THE CRAZY BOOKWORM

BOOKS, MENTAL HEALTH AND ME

BECKY POWELL

CONTENTS

A little note from me in 2021 ix

Chapter 1	1
Chapter 2	5
Chapter 3	9
Chapter 4	13
Chapter 5	17
Chapter 6	21
Chapter 7	25
Chapter 8	31
Chapter 9	37
Chapter 10	41
Chapter 11	45
Chapter 12	49
Chapter 13	55
Chapter 14	63
Chapter 15	69
Chapter 16	73
Chapter 17	79
Chapter 18	83
Chapter 19	89
Chapter 20	95
Chapter 21	99
Chapter 22	103
Chapter 23	107
Chapter 24	111
Chapter 25	115
Chapter 26	121
Chapter 27	125
Chapter 28	131
Chapter 29	137
Chapter 30	143
Chapter 31	147

The Comfort Tree	149
Bibliography	151

For Archie x

"A room without books is like a body without a soul."
- Louisa May Alcott, *Little Women.*

A LITTLE NOTE FROM ME IN 2021

Hello Reader,

I guess that if you are reading these words then I finally got round to writing my story.

Five years ago I experienced a mental breakdown and was diagnosed with severe depression and anxiety. I struggled to function, leave the house, or even get the rubbish bins in from wherever the dustmen had decided to leave them. But I was one of the lucky ones because during that awful time I had a lovely husband, family and friends to support me. Many people have no one and have to struggle alone.

I found that journaling and reading my treasured books helped my recovery. It enabled me to reflect and try to understand what had happened for me to reach this point. I guess the written word helped me to move forward. I still have my own mental health challenges, but I have learnt to manage them better.

Books have always been part of my DNA; without them I feel unanchored from myself. Here I share some of the wonderful books that are dear to me.

Now we are all living through the COVID 19 pandemic, and mental health is more important than ever. Unfortunately, it continues to be greatly misunderstood and not talked about nearly enough. I hope this book inspires and comforts you enough to know that you are not alone.

I stumbled upon a quote recently by Annie Dillard: *she read books as one would breathe air, to fill up and live*. For me, books aren't just things to pass the time when it's raining outside and the television schedule offers little entertainment. They are happy endings I can aspire to, and worlds I can get lost in. They help me feel complete.

Within the beauty of those pages is a place where anything is possible.

Enjoy. X

CHAPTER 1

My lovely grandma, books and me

"A house needs a grandma in it."
- Louisa May Alcott

My grandma worked hard. She had a big garden where she grew all her own vegetables and herbs. I have many memories of her knee-deep in the vegetable patch picking potatoes for tea, dirt on her knees and hands. As always, she was wearing her apron and the pockets were brimming full of potatoes. She would have a handful of homegrown mint clutched in her coarse hands (they were hands that worked hard) ready to add to the potatoes; it always set them apart from the ones my mum fed me.

Grandma lived in the countryside and her garden backed onto a park that led onto fields. We would go for endless picnics and walks over those fields, picking blackberries that stained our fingers. We would hurry back full of excitement and Grandma would magic them into a delicious fruit crumble together with apples picked from her tree.

She was nice, my grandma, not affectionate or loving but solid and dependable, as was the case with people from her generation. The best thing about staying at her house, aside from the delicious food, were the books that I could read and the stories that I wrote when I was there.

I spent a lot of time on my own when I was growing up as both my sisters were significantly older. I enjoyed being on my own, though, and I found a companion in books and putting pen to paper. I could often be found sitting in the park reading a book that I had taken off the dusty bookshelf. I loved that unique smell of the musty pages and would frequently hold the books to my nose and inhale their pungent odour. It made me feel happy.

I had a special Toby jug on a shelf by the fire that held all my pencils and pens. Securely placed underneath was a pile of paper that my grandma kept for me to write on. I made up endless stories and turned them into little books, with front covers that I designed carefully with my coloured pencils. No one ever read my books, only me. I didn't think they were very good but, nonetheless, I enjoyed the process.

Another thing I loved was the real fire Grandma always had, which meant we could toast marshmallows and crumpets speared on the ends of sticks. I adored biting through the caramelised outer skin of the marshmallows to taste the sweet, sticky, middle bit that melted on my tongue. After filling up on whatever delightful food she gave me, I would sit quietly by the fire and write stories of made-up lands and adventures.

I used to pretend I was Darrell Rivers from the Malory Towers books by Enid Blyton, which I loved reading when I was young. They told the adventures of Darrell and her friends who attended an all-girls' boarding school. I would often lose myself in writing about a girl who could do anything and was popular. Sometimes my grandma's front room was filled with people – my parents, my sisters or other relatives. It would get very noisy on occasion but I would continue to sit quietly, lost in the world of a book that I was reading or a story I was writing.

I was often described as quiet and shy when I was young, which I didn't really like because I felt it wasn't necessarily a good thing to be. Consequently, the fictitious world of the books took on an even stronger meaning and became a haven, enabling me to believe that I could be anything. In that world I could achieve anything with no questions asked. When I was lost in the words I felt alive, vivid. I felt that I was no longer invisible, which was a real comfort. That was the best thing of all.

CHAPTER 2

Little old me in 2015

"Me, myself and I."
- J.D.Salinger, *The Catcher in the Rye*

I once asked my husband to try to describe me in three words. He said I was kind, hard-working and dizzy. I would agree with that. Other people often describe me as bubbly; I always smile because it makes me sound like a sparkling wine.

One thing I know about myself is that I need things to aim for. The greater the challenge, the better. For example, I completed an English degree whilst working full time as a nurse, and I trained for the London Marathon whilst raising a significant sum of money for charity.

I am fiercely loyal and a perfectionist. I love with all my heart, and I know that I expect a lot from people. I am strong-willed and strong-minded, which is not always a good thing, but it runs in our family.

I am also a person filled with self-doubt and feelings of never quite being good enough. Even my achievements only offer me a small amount of pleasure for a short time, then I default back to feeling worthless.

What else about me? Well, I live with a lovely caring husband, a nine-year-old son and two cats. I have a good job and no real money issues. I live in a safe area with friendly neighbours. I have a small but very close circle of friends. I like the theatre, reading and socialising. I love animals and I am partial to a cocktail or two. I am forty-four years old, tall, blonde and decent looking. I guess you could describe me as just your average Jo Bloggs.

I have had difficulties, as most of us do, but I have had my fair share of happy times as well. I suppose it is only human nature to want to hold onto those happy moments and experience them constantly, but life isn't like that. Happiness is a fleeting emotion, just like any other.

For someone like me, it is that realisation that is so painful. When I feel sad and life is challenging, it is like a huge dark cloud has settled around me. Although things may improve and that fleeting happy feeling returns, the dark cloud always remains close by. There can be momentary breaks in it that offers some light, but the darkness is always the dominant force.

I think that is why I try to stay busy, filling my life with challenges, trying to stay one step ahead of the darkness in my mind that has the potential to consume it at any moment. The effort of always trying to outmanoeuvre those feelings is exhausting, and I guess there had to be a limit to how long I could continue to do it.

I can't recall the exact moment that the darkness caught up with me and my thought patterns started to shift dramatically. At first it was a niggle, like a tiny crack in a vase that you don't notice as long as you don't focus on it for too long. But as the days passed, I started to notice it more. It was the feeling of fear, worthlessness and impending doom. I was really scared of what was going to happen.

During those days, I kept recalling my dad's words when he knew he was going to die. He said that he felt he hadn't done a lot with his life, and that made me so incredibly sad. I became blindingly aware of my own lack of achievements, how the years were ticking by and I still felt like life was a struggle. I felt worthless.

Very quickly those feelings began to consume my every hour, every minute, every second. Then one day the tiny crack shattered the vase into a million pieces. My brain experienced a severe chemical imbalance … and my whole world tipped on its side.

CHAPTER 3

April 2015
The day of reckoning

"There may be no light at the end of the tunnel ... you must keep going, because that is your duty."
- Mani Ashwin

It seems that I have entered a long, dark tunnel. I feel scared, hopeless and alone. How did I get here? The life I was once part of has vanished. It is so confusing because I was on the train of life, moving along quite happily but now it seems that I'm not. I'm in this tunnel and the darkness is like a lethal injection that has entered my body, powerfully flowing through my veins, suffocating me with every painful breath.

If I could just get out of this tunnel, there it will be – my life, waiting impatiently for me at the next station. Ignoring the menacing voice in my head is useless. I try with all the strength I can summon to find a way out.

Surely there has to be some light in the tunnel? I can hear the voice again answering impatiently, as if I am stupid, 'Yes, of course there is light – it will be at the end. It's only a tunnel, so the daylight is somewhere.'

I realise I have been so silly. I just have to keep going, and I will eventually see the light and that will guide me out. For a moment I feel a glimmer of comfort. I should know there is always an end to everything: a beginning and an end. The end always feels hopeful because it is in the future and hasn't happened yet.

But then I hear the voice saying a little louder that there is no end to this tunnel. There is no light and there is no way out.

The screaming inside my head won't stop because I know the voice is right. I just haven't wanted to believe it until now. In a way, believing it brings some relief.

I realise that I need help.

I make it to the doctor's, but I can't remember how I got here. I sit in the waiting room, looking at my fellow patients in a daze. I want to leave so badly. I can feel people looking at me and I can hear them thinking, 'She looks healthy enough, so why is she here?' The waiting is agony: thirty, long, painful minutes.

I sit opposite the doctor and can taste salt in my mouth. I realise it's the taste of the tears rolling down my face. The doctor looks concerned, and I think that she has a nice, kind face. I try to articulate how I feel but it is impossible. If I could just write all my feelings down on the pad on her desk then they would make sense to her. She would understand my hopelessness, loneliness, isolation, fear and deep-rooted sorrow completely.

I must have made her understand in some way because she offers me a prescription. I clutch it tightly in my hand as I stumble clumsily out of the building into the daylight. The solution: 20mg of Fluoxetine once a day.

For a while this seems to work but then, six months later, I experience a revelation. I wake up one fine day and realise that my path in life is always going to be a struggle. I may always have this feeling that happiness, success, money, luck happen to other people. People's lives are good and sometimes not so good, but they seem to change, grow and evolve in a way that enriches them, in a way that mine seems not to. It makes me question what I did wrong in a previous life.

CHAPTER 4

Mad, me?

"You're mad, bonkers. Completely off your head. But I'll tell you a secret. All the best people are."
- Lewis Carroll, *Alice in Wonderland*

I wake in the middle of the night covered in sweat and check the time on my phone. It reads 2.50am. My husband is next to me, sleeping deeply and snoring without a care in the world. Going back to sleep would be a futile exercise so I lie there in the darkness, staring unblinking into the void. The only sound is the tick of the landing clock and the erratic beat of my heart. They seem to be in competition with each other as to which one can be the loudest.

The hands of the clock eventually get to seven o'clock and it is my time to get up. I know I can't go to work today. My husband won't know this because I get dressed and do my hair and make-up. I still look like me: immaculate. But inside I am dying.

He has no idea that I have been taking medication for six months. He has been living with someone with depression for months and hasn't noticed anything at all, such has been my ability to mask the storm raging inside me. I have been sinking like a stone, but everything has appeared normal. The house has been cleaned, our son has been looked after, my husband's work shirts have been ironed every Sunday, ready for the week ahead. My world, however, has been spiralling out of control. Thoughts of worthlessness and an impending sense of doom have consumed me, packed inside me so tightly that I feel like I can't breathe.

I drive my son to school and drop him off safely at the school gates. Returning home, my mind is foggy as I grip the steering wheel. If I speed up and drive into the lorry in front of me, all of this will be over. Then I think of my son and my mum, and I come to my senses. I hear my late father's voice in my ear. 'You can get through this,' he tells me.

I spend most of the day (aside from a failed attempt at going for a walk) lying on the bed looking out of the window at the bare trees. I only get up when it is time to collect my son from school. He manages to put a smile on my face with important questions such as, 'What sponsor of crisps are your favourite?' He means brand and flavour.

'Walker's prawn cocktail,' I tell him.

He looks at me for a moment and then says, 'Yeuch!'

My husband comes home from work, takes one look at me and describes me as a complete zombie. In a small way that makes me feel vindicated because it is true that I have no idea what is going on around me at the moment. He gently asks me to describe my day and I have to refrain from laughing because my day hasn't consisted of anything. I recall there was a drive back from school where I contemplated suicide, but if someone told me I had driven two hundred miles I wouldn't have argued with them. This was followed by a failed attempt to go for a walk to post my sister's birthday card. I couldn't make it halfway down the road before having to run, breathless, back to the safety of our four walls. I tell him that the effort of posting that card would be like someone telling me to walk to Edinburgh to post it. Totally unthinkable.

He tries to get me to eat something. My response is a cutting, 'You can't bloody make me. I'll go and have a bath.'

Afterwards, I come downstairs and can't remember that I've had a bath until I feel my wet hair dripping on my neck and look down at my dressing gown. I sit on the edge of the sofa and it feels strange. As I feel the water running down my back, I have no idea what I am supposed to do next.

My husband tells me, 'You've had a mental breakdown.'

The following morning, he rings work to tell them he won't be coming in. It makes me feel bad about myself. As I lie on the bed I can hear him on the phone to the doctor's surgery making an appointment for me. I have no idea how I am going to bear leaving the house.

The appointment is at 11.20am and my husband supports me as I get in the car and out at the other end. I sit there for ages, willing myself to move but not being able to because I know there will be another long wait in the waiting room with all eyes on me. Then I think of my son and know I have to try.

The GP thinks I will benefit from some counselling and cognitive behavioural therapy, and she recommends a charity based in the city centre called the Link. The waiting list is about three weeks which, in my present state, feel like an eternity away. I start to cry.

The doctor grabs my hand then asks me gently, 'When was the last time you felt right?'

I have no idea how to answer this question and think to myself, *Never, I would say.* But that doesn't seem acceptable so instead I pluck a number out of the air. 'Four or five months,' I tell her.

'And have you ever thought about harming yourself?' she asks.

I glance anxiously at my husband, who looks overwhelmed. I feel the small cuts on my legs itching beneath my jeans. It's as if they are saying, 'Trying to hide us won't help you in the end.' The cutting makes me feel alive in some way, helps me to know that I do exist, but because I have only made a few it hardly seems relevant to mention them.

'No,' I lie.

The doctor diagnoses me with severe depression and anxiety. As she says those words they sound distant and unnatural, as if she is speaking them to someone else.

At home, my husband cries. He tells me that 'he is having a moment'. He says that it is so hard seeing me like this, but I have no capacity to take on his feelings.

I say, 'You have caused this in some way.' I clearly want to hurt the person closest to me.

'I know,' he replies.

CHAPTER 5

The dreaded D word

"There are wounds that never show on the body that are deeper and more hurtful than anything that bleeds."
- Laurel K. Hamilton, *Mistral's Kiss*

The *Oxford Dictionary* defines depression as '*a pathological state of extreme dejection or melancholy often with physical symptoms, a reduction in vitality, vigour or spirits*'.

I put the dictionary to one side. Nineteen words to describe the feelings of pain and hopelessness that sweep through your body like an unstoppable wave crashing onto rocks. They don't come close to conveying those feelings.

I remember from my nursing studies that the part of the brain called the hippocampus is important in terms of depression because it is an area of the brain in the temporal lobe involved with long-term memory, forming new memories and connecting emotions to those memories. I always used to call it 'the hippopotamus'. I think I said to one of my nursing friends that it made me think of a bunch of hippies camping. We probably found it amusing when we were aged nineteen.

On *The Guardian* website I find an article written by Melissa Davey that highlights the importance of treating depression early.

Fifteen research institutes around the world collaborated their studies comparing the hippocampus of depressed and healthy people. They examined the brain magnetic resonance imaging data of 8.927 people, 1,728 of whom had major depression and the rest of whom were healthy. The researchers found 65% of the depressed study participants had recurrent depression and it was these people who had a smaller hippocampus.

The article goes onto say that there is good evidence that the damage is reversible with treatment. This is because the hippocampus is one of the unique areas of the brain that can rapidly generate new connections between cells. It says that social interventions are just as important as taking medication, but there is some evidence that the hippocampus is larger in those patients taking antidepressants. This would indicate the protective effect of these tablets. I feel a tiny wave of comfort knowing that the medication will help me.

I also have a look on the NHS website www.nhs.uk which contains a wealth of information on mental health. As I have been diagnosed with severe depression I identify immediately with the symptoms I am experiencing:

- Low self-esteem
- Feeling guilt ridden
- Not getting any enjoyment out of life

- Feeling anxious or worried
- Disturbed sleep
- Changes in appetite
- Lack of energy

The treatment for severe depression is a combination therapy of antidepressants and cognitive behavioural therapy. Having both together is more effective.

Anxiety has accompanied my depression, rather like an annoying sibling. This is quite common. Again there is a long list of symptoms of which mine include:

- Restlessness
- Tiredness
- Dizziness
- Pins and needles
- Insomnia: difficulty falling or staying asleep
- Dry mouth
- Trembling or shaking

The treatment for anxiety is cognitive behavioural therapy first, then medication if the therapy doesn't work on its own.

But despite all the evidence and research, it seems that understanding the true causes of depression and anxiety is still somewhat rudimentary. Looking on the King's Fund website, I learn that three in four people with a mental health problem in England receive little or no treatment for their condition. There are large gaps in terms of health outcomes because people with the most severe mental illnesses die on average fifteen to twenty years earlier than the general population. Mental health problems account for 23% of the burden of disease in the UK, but spending on mental health services consumes only 11% of the NHS budget.

It makes for very bleak reading and leaves me feeling hopeless. I wonder how I am going to get better. It seems like I am looking at a mountain I have to climb whose summit is completely hidden by clouds. The thought of even trying leaves me scared and exhausted.

As I stare at the bare trees moving in the wind, I reflect on my internet research. There is no mention of the one thing that is so important when describing depression – that it is invisible.

CHAPTER 6

Do the drugs work?

"I have absolutely no pleasure in stimulants in which I sometimes so madly indulge ... it has been the desperate attempt to escape from torturing memories ... and a dread of some strange impending doom."
- Edgar Allan Poe

A long with the information about the counselling service, the GP has given me another prescription for antidepressants. This time it's Sertraline 25mg for one week and then an increase to 50mg daily. It seems a high dose to me, but the doctor has told me it isn't. She has also given me sleeping tablets, Zopiclone 7.5mg, as I told her I wasn't sleeping. The doctor told me in a voice like a teacher, 'They can be addictive, so can't be taken for very long.' Always the good student, I will do as I'm told.

My husband collects the prescription straight away and I think to myself, *It must be serious, then.*

He takes me for a walk; he thinks it would be good for me to get some fresh air. We get as far as the end of our road before I can't get my breath and my surroundings seem to close in on me. I have to get home to be safe, into my little cocoon that protects me from life where I can lie on my bed and look out at the tops of the bare trees.

I take a sleeping tablet that night. I fall asleep quickly and sleep deeply. I dream of trees attacking me and throwing apples at me. My grandma's face morphs into the Wicked Witch of the West from *The Wizard of Oz*.

As I take the tablets over the coming days, I start to look forward to taking the Zopiclone and religiously watch the hands of the clock move towards eight o'clock. I don't know specifically why that time, but it becomes part of my routine. It takes around thirty to forty-five minutes before my eyelids start to feel heavy. The effort required to keep them open is like attempting to not blink for twenty-four hours. As soon as I start experiencing the weightlessness in my limbs, I feel a surge of pleasure because I know that soon I will not have to feel anything. I can understand why they are addictive.

The following day, I often wake up with a head that feels like someone has stuffed it full of cotton wool. I have a metallic taste in my dry mouth and a day of feeling sleepy ahead of me. I read on the leaflet in the box that these are common side effects.

I can feel the growth in my brain possessing me today, and I fear the outcome will be grim. I have started taking my Sertraline. I was told by my doctor it is used in the treatment of depression by increasing the levels of serotonin in the brain. Serotonin is a neurotransmitter that is thought to have a good influence on mood and emotions.

The side effects from this drug, which I am suffering from, are:

- Difficulty in sleeping
- Dizziness
- Headache
- Nausea
- Dry mouth
- Tiredness
- Increase sweating
- Grinding of teeth
- Nightmares
- Upset stomach
- Anxiety
- Feeling strange

These are all mentioned in the patient information leaflet. Just reading it increases my anxiety and makes my mouth drier so I throw the leaflet in the bin. But, despite all their side effects, I know I need them. Hopefully they will give me that little bit of strength to see more clearly the light at the end of the tunnel. I also know that taking these tablets alone is sticking a plaster over a gaping wound; it's only masking the problem, not healing it.

I go upstairs for a lie down and open my bedside drawer to check my tablets are all safely stored. Next to the all-too-obvious medication is my pink notebook that I keep there to record random thoughts and reminders of things that need doing.

I take it out, open it and turn the crisp pages. It is empty apart from a few shopping lists. When was the last time I wrote anything? Trying to remember makes my head feel foggy again.

I remember writing journals during my travels in Australia and when my mum was battling cancer. The journal writing has always been a comfort, but I haven't written anything in so long.

I try to think when I last read a book. Everything is so upside down and inside out at the moment. The tangible feel of a favourite book in my hand feels like a comforting but distant memory. My fingers twitch emptily, knowing that I need my books again.

My head is pounding as I close the drawer. When I was a naive eighteen year old, I announced to my family with all the confidence of youth that I wanted to be a published writer. That Christmas, my sister and brother-in-law bought me a beautiful William Morris notebook. I remember that I loved the design of the cover; it was all blues, pinks and greens.

I told them that I would write my book and be a successful writer. I remember my sister saying to me, 'Well, I hope you do it.' My dad had enjoyed recording us on his new video camera that year, so my words were immortalised forever. I can watch the recording anytime and reflect on the hopeful, dream-filled eighteen year old that I was. I feel sad that I never did fill those pages with my book.

I open the drawer again, take out my current pink-covered notebook and lie down on the bed with it resting next to me. I close my eyes. Soon my son will be home from school.

I only have four hours to wait.

CHAPTER 7

The saviour of books

"I had always found that being alone was not good ... but my books were always my friends."
- Joshua Slocum, *Sailing Alone around the World*

A new week. When I wake up this morning, I have the same nasty taste in my mouth. *Something is rotten in the state of Denmark.*

My husband brings me a cup of tea in bed. 'You have to get up,' he tells me.

'Why?' I ask.

'Because if you don't get up now, then you won't get up at all.'

I do it, even though I hate him for it.

I seem to have fallen into a routine. I get up and get dressed, usually in the clothes that I discarded on the bedroom chair the night before. This makes it easier for me in the mornings because I don't have to stand looking at my clothes in hopeless bewilderment, wondering what to put on. No make up; the old me wore make up virtually every day, regardless.

I spray myself with my husband's aftershave, which is a bit odd but it gives me comfort. I think it's because I don't want to smell like me at the moment because that feels wrong somehow. I tie my hair back in a ponytail and put a grip either side. I make our bed, then make our son's bed and attempt to tidy the pile of cuddly toys that keep him company when he is asleep. Somehow they seem to multiply during the night.

I venture downstairs, unload the dishwasher and wash up the breakfast dishes that my son and husband have left. These have to be washed, dried and put away. I don't really know why I don't put them in the dishwasher, but I think it's the idea of them sitting in there all day, dirty and unloved.

I feed the cats. I get out six pouches and lay them on the kitchen work surface in two lines of three. I am having to ration them because the ginger one, Sheamus, would eat all day long if he could. The vet has already told me he shouldn't get any bigger. This is incredibly hard when Sheamus looks up at me with those round, kind eyes.

My husband and son get ready to leave. My son has his rucksack with his homework done and a snack inside, and he is wearing his warm coat. He is my reason to want to get better.

My husband asks me, 'Are you going to be alright today? What are you going to do?' He looks completely baffled when I tell him that I have decided to do some writing and reading. I'm hoping the words will help me make sense of why I got to this point. Maybe it will help me *regain some vigour and strength* as the *Oxford Dictionary* says, although I am not convinced I had either of those attributes to begin with.

My husband seems completely lost. 'I don't get it. I don't know how that is going to help you.' He tells me that I should look at some form of meditation.

I know that he has my best interests at heart, and maybe in time I would benefit from some form of relaxation therapy, but right now scribbling thoughts down in my notebook and leafing through the well-worn pages of my books seems like the right thing to do. I need to be in my happy place again. I crave something more than taking tablets.

I remember reading once about a woman who had terminal cancer. She had always loved writing and she started writing every morning. Gradually, as the days passed, she began to get excited about the characters and the story she was creating. Very soon she was focusing on her writing instead of the pain that was engulfing her body. She got a dog as well, something to keep her company, a living thing that needed her.

When the house is empty and everyone has departed, gone to wherever they need to be for the day, I have my two cats. Sheamus is the big fat ginger one; my son named him after his favourite WWE wrestler. Cleo is black and grey, and has black circling her eyes like eyeliner, like Cleopatra. They are very good at keeping me company. I have them, my pink notebook and my books.

The sofa is beckoning today, and the trees and birds are waiting for me to stare glassily at them. A little robin is hopping around the branches, looking so free and happy. I look at my many books on the bookshelf and my glance falls on *I Know why the Caged Bird Sings* by Maya Angelou.

I first read this book aged twenty-six, as part of my English Literature degree. I have always loved the title, which apparently Angelou took from a favourite poet of hers, Paul Lawrence Dunbar. I guess the caged bird sings because he has lost his freedom and it is his way of being able to endure the bars around him. Maybe he still feels hope. I wish I could have that feeling where hopelessness is replaced by hopeful. I take the book, open it and inhale the pages.

The book is Angelou's autobiographical account of growing up as a black African American. The memoir tells the story of her traumatic childhood where she endures rape and racism, and struggles to find her place in the world. *'If growing up is painful for the Southern Black girl, being aware of her displacement is the rust on the razor that threatens the throat. It is an unnecessary insult.'*

It is the displacement that depression can often bring which is hard to deal with. I am painfully aware of my illness and how I am detached from the rest of the world. The people I know go to work, school, shopping, etc., and I feel like a failure as I am unable to do these things at the moment. As the world around me continues to turn, I stand alone, so far removed from it . There is me, and then there is everyone else looking on, judging me for my disfigured brain.

The one thing in the book that always pulls at my heartstrings is Angelou's sheer will to survive the most brutal events. When I first read this book, I had just lost my lovely dad to cancer and my studying enabled me to keep my mind focused on something other than my grief. When I read the account of the rape Angelou suffered at the hands of Mr Freeman, her mother's boyfriend, I cried. She was only eight years old. It was the first time I had cried over something that wasn't to do with losing my dad.

Angelou's trauma caused her to go mute. A friend, Mrs Bertha Flowers, was the person who got her to speak again. She explained the importance of not only reading but speaking the words out loud to bring them to life, and gave Angelou books for this purpose.

Mrs Flowers was an important figure in Angelou's life. Despite not mentoring her for long, it was enough to reignite Angelou's love of books. Angelou writes: *'I wouldn't miss Mrs Flowers, because she had given me her secret word which called forth a dijinn who was to serve me all my life: books.'*

This is the other reason I adore this book: I can relate to Angelou's love of books. For me, they are the sum of all parts. Whenever I have felt lost in my life, I just have to start reading a book I love and suddenly it's like finding a missing piece of a puzzle. The picture starts to become clearer.

Trying to cope with mental illness is a constant battle. You don't want to be like you are, but you can't see a way out. Turning to something where you find joy can be the ointment that soothes. It might be books, or it might be something completely different, maybe cooking, painting, pottery or something else entirely. It doesn't matter as long as it lights up your soul.

Find it and hold onto it firmly while the waves crash around you. Maybe it will help the waters to calm for a while.

CHAPTER 8

Green fingers are good

"I like gardening. It's a place where *I can find myself when I need to lose myself."*
- Alice Seabold

This morning, as I am scribbling some of my thoughts in my pink notebook, I am sitting on the sofa in the lounge looking at the trees and watching the birds dancing through the branches.

I receive a text from one of my friends. It seems mental illness really is all around us. She says that she's had depression for almost a year and applauds the fact that I am up and dressed. It is an achievement. *That is only because my husband makes me,* I think. If it was down to me, I would still be under the duvet hiding from the world.

What have you told them at work? my friend texts.

I just told them it's personal issues, I text back.

Keep it that way as there's a lot of stigma with depression.

I reflect on her words. If she had been diagnosed with cancer, people would be rallying around, literally tripping over each other to help. They would be baking cakes, raising money and even shaving their heads. The human mind is completely misunderstood but, like any other organ in the body, it can degenerate and mutate. I feel mine rotting inside my skull.

Another text comes through from my husband: Where are you?

Momentarily I wonder if I'm supposed to be somewhere else. At home! I text back.

He tells me to go to the MIND website as it may be worthwhile. I know he is trying to help me, but it is incredibly tiring having to do these things.

I'll see if I can, I text back.

***

I quickly send a text to my friend to ask her if she would pick my son up from school. I tell her I have a migraine. It's easier that way.

MIND: The mental health charity www.mind.org.uk

Their ethos:

We provide advice and support to empower anyone experiencing a mental health problem. We campaign to improve services, raise awareness and promote understanding.

We won't give up until everyone experiencing a mental health problem gets support and respect.

I read that one in four people in any given year experience mental health problems. I had no idea that it was such a high figure. All of those people are experiencing this awful condition, a real condition just like any other. Not something that is made up or should be hidden away, not something to feel guilty or embarrassed about. Will these people get better or not? Or will they just have to live with their condition and try to manage it as best they can?

The MIND website offers advice, support and guidance. Being a keen gardener I am particularly drawn to two of their programmes.

ECOTHERAPY PROGRAMMES:

A trained therapist leads you through different activities to develop a balanced relationship with nature that benefits your well-being which often includes cognitive behavioural therapy.

WEEKLY GREEN GYMS:

General garden activities as well as construction of community gardens. There is one located in Birmingham, which isn't that far from where I live, within a housing complex which is currently overgrown and unloved. It will become a food growing space and access for all residents.

I don't know why, but I send them an email to ask about getting involved. I love the idea of the project, clearing an unused space and making it into something beautiful, a space for people whose lives haven't turned out like they thought they would. Hope is all they have, and maybe an area of peaceful nature to enjoy will keep that hope alive.

I am lucky that I have wonderful family and friends to support me. Some people have nobody to turn to when their lives fall apart.

The restorative feeling that gardening can give, and its help in combatting depression, is well documented. I used to own an allotment where I grew loads of different vegetables and flowers. I remember the first things I ever grew were potatoes because all of the books I read said they were an easy thing to start with. When I dug out my first potato, it was like digging out a beautiful, rare jewel. I felt a mixture of surprise and elation as I held it in my hand.

I also grew tomatoes very successfully and they became one of my favourites. Like the books say, the smell can always lift my spirits; it is supposed to release endorphins. I made some of the tomatoes into relishes and chutneys, put them into little jars and handed them into the eager hands of family and friends. I remember that, momentarily, it made me feel good about myself.

I used to love sitting down in the allotment on a summer's day, drinking my mug of tea and chatting to my fellow workers. When you own an allotment and are growing various crops, it makes you very aware of the seasons. My favourite season is autumn because it brings an intensity to all of the senses. I love the russets and golds, and the glorious smell of the leaves as they crunch underfoot. The simple pleasure of sitting down in an allotment, feeling the sun on your face and the smell of earth on your fingers, undoubtedly enriches the soul. In those moments I thought more about what I was creating around me than about myself and, temporarily, I experienced some relief.

Of course, in my present state the idea that I can drive all the way to Birmingham (some twenty miles) and participate in the programme is ridiculous. Some might say I have more chance of landing on the moon.

CHAPTER 9

It's what's inside that really counts

"Your will shall decide your destiny."
- Charlotte Brontë, *Jane Eyre*

My husband watches intently as I swallow my 50mg Sertraline tablet with the cup of tea he has brought me. He seems satisfied with this. I notice he is dressed in Lycra, which tells me he must be going out on his bike. He has the day off today and chooses to spend it this way. He will be gone for hours. There could be an earthquake happening and he would still get on his bike.

'You don't mind me doing this today, do you?' he asks.

How can I respond to that? Part of me is glad that he is going because I know it will do him good and it also gives me time to get on with my writing. I know I won't be ironing his shirts for work any time soon. Not one single one. I am enjoying the process of writing – if I'm totally honest, more than enjoying it. It helps me get through the day until my son returns from school.

I was re-reading *Jane Eyre* before my 'breakdown', but it now lies discarded in my bedside drawer. Today I get it out and look at it. The spine of the book is broken, and the front page is creased and has a tea stain on it. There are parts of the text underlined with little notes scribbled next to them; I studied this book for my dissertation. This is Charlotte Brontë's most famous novel and my favourite of hers. As I read the opening line, '*There was no possibility of taking a walk that day,*' I smile to myself. At the moment, due to my agoraphobia, there is no possibility of my taking a walk today or any day!

My intention on re-reading *Jane Eyre* was to do it for pleasure alone. In some ways it is similar to Maya Angelou's book: it is a story of a woman who has to face many challenges in her life and find a way to overcome them. Jane Eyre is a girl who is tiny of stature but has an enormous spirit and heart. She endures life's challenges and succeeds.

Everyone's experience of depression is unique, and how they learn to deal with it is very different. At this moment, as I battle my demons, I know that most of what will happen to me going forward will depend on my inner strength. My future will be determined by how much I desire to get better and my willingness to take help from any available source. I can't rely on anyone else to change my life, it is down to me. I think to myself that if only there were a better version of myself that existed then I might stand a chance.

Jane Eyre begins with Jane's life with the Reeds' family. She is an orphan and her kind uncle sends for her, but unfortunately he dies before she arrives. The Reeds' household is not a happy place for Jane, and she is bullied by her cousins and abused by her aunt.

She is locked in the Red Room where her late uncle died and she faints when she thinks she sees his ghost.

The next part of Jane's journey takes her to Lowood Boarding School, a cold and ghastly place. The teachers are mostly cruel, and the pupils are always freezing cold and hungry. Jane has to endure the death of her dear friend, Helen Burns, from consumption. It is only when Jane arrives at Thornfield Hall and meets the mysterious Mr Rochester that there is a glimmer of happiness for her.

Eventually they fall in love and he proposes marriage. But Mr Rochester has a secret: he is already married to Bertha Mason, the *mad woman* who is locked away from view in the attic. I always had a vivid imagination as a child and had nightmares of witches in my wardrobe, goblins under my bed and clothes moving on the back of my bedroom door, so this woman lurking in the attic, pacing the floor and laughing both frightened me and captivated my imagination.

Thankfully, Jane does get her happy ending: '*Reader, I married him.*' Whenever I finish reading this book, it leaves me comforted and hopeful. If Jane can succeed through all of her hardships and be rewarded with her happy ending, then maybe I will be too. If I can just try to keep going, maybe there it will be just around the corner – my rainbow with a pot of gold at the end.

CHAPTER 10

Those people in white coats

"Doctors?" said Ron, looking startled. "Those Muggle nutters that cut people up?"
- J.K.Rowling, *Harry Potter and the Order of the Phoenix*

My husband returns from work this morning to take me to my doctor's appointment. Hopefully the doctor won't suggest ECT or putting me into a straitjacket. I think of Jack Nicholson in *One Flew over the Cuckoo's Nest* and I am really hoping that she won't say, 'Mrs Powell, a complete lobotomy is needed. I'm afraid it's the only answer.'

I have to be supported by my husband as I walk to the car, and also at the other end into the doctor's waiting room. I don't want to get out of the passenger seat but somehow I manage to.

I take thirty-two excruciating steps in total. When eventually I am sitting in front of the doctor, I see something beneath her kind expression: doubt. Doesn't she believe me? I try and tell myself that I am being paranoid, but I can't shake the feeling and it sort of makes me give up.

The doctor tells me that the only way I can see a counsellor in less than three weeks is if she contacts the crisis team, and she can only do that if I've planned to put measures in place to kill myself. 'Have you done that?' She asks me this like she is asking me what my favourite food is.

Instead of replying with sweet-and-sour chicken, I tell her that no, I haven't actually planned how I am going to end it all. So thankfully, it looks like my admittance to a psychiatric ward followed by a lobotomy isn't going to happen just yet.

The doctor asks me what I've eaten today. 'Half a piece of toast,' I tell her, which makes her frown.

'And drinking?' she asks.

I want to say, 'Oh, you know – gin, vodka, whisky – it depends on my mood.' But I don't, of course. 'Water and decaffeinated tea,' I tell her.

She seems pleased with this.

'My husband won't let me have caffeine.' I say this with an undercurrent of resentment.

Later I feel that the doctor would be pleased because when I get back home I consume a three-course meal.

- Starter: 4 x melon squares; 2 x kiwi squares; a handful of redcurrants; a handful of blueberries.
- Main course: 4 x sticks of asparagus wrapped in two pieces of chorizo.
- Dessert: 1 x chocolate biscuit.

Surely I must be getting better?

I feel exhausted now. Time to lie down.

That evening I receive an email from MIND about conservation volunteering. Tom, the organiser, tells me that there are plenty of projects going on in the Birmingham area and it would be great if I could join them.

I will have to email him and say that, due to my inability to leave the house, it will be impossible for me to attend. Or as my faithful *Oxford Dictionary* describes it:

Agoraphobia: an abnormal fear of open spaces or public spaces.

If only it were as simple as that description.

I notice that the dustmen have collected the rubbish, and the bins are at the end of the drive. How many steps to the bin and back, I wonder?

I am not going to find out.

CHAPTER 11

To err is human

"If you know someone who's depressed, please resolve never to ask them why. Depression isn't a straightforward response to a bad situation; depression just is, like the weather."
- Stephen Fry

The following morning, my husband brings me a cup of tea (decaffeinated) and tells me that I must not forget to take my antidepressant. I wonder if he's been in my drawer, counting the tablets. I know he wants me to be well again, but I just hope he realises it isn't going to be a quick process.

I seem to have fallen into a routine in the mornings. Following my daily activities (short, I know!) I sit on the sofa. This has to be by 8.30am or I start feeling anxious. Then I start my writing.

I like sitting here in the lounge with one of the cats somewhere close by. I can look out of the window and see people walking their dogs, cars arriving and going to work, and people carrying out simple everyday errands. Do they take their health for granted, I wonder?

My phone pings with a text message from a friend: How are you doing? Hope you are doing ok!!!

It's the three exclamation marks that wound.

Since this all started, I have received many texts from friends and family saying that they are here for me, and if there is anything I need to just ask. How do I do that, I wonder? The last thing I can manage is to ask them for help. It is impossible to articulate how I am feeling, and I fear it would come across as quite lame and pathetic. People would think, 'Oh for goodness' sake, is that all it is?'

Here are some examples of what people have said since my illness began.

'Boy, you look better. I don't really understand all this, but I think it's like taking baby steps. Setting small targets. Maybe try walking to the end of the road and back.'

<u>My thoughts:</u> If only he knew that it would be like trying to climb Mount Everest without training or equipment – totally impossible.

I know I will struggle to put the recycling out today. I probably won't do it. I think about putting on the TV but won't; I like the idea of it, but I know I won't be able to. If I didn't have my husband and son to keep going for I would undoubtedly just stop, crawl back into bed and hide under the duvet. As Shakespeare writes in *Macbeth*: *'her eyes are open... but their sense is shut.'* Most definitely.

'I am keeping my fingers crossed that you return to your former self!!!'

My thoughts: Maybe the exclamation marks affirm that a return to my former self with all of my issues would be a bad thing. Anyway, I don't want to because my old self got me here in the first place. My husband has said to me, which was nice, 'You will be you again, but a stronger, better version of yourself.'

'I mean, what actually is depression?'

My thoughts: I hope you never find out.

'I am praying for you.'

My thoughts: I'm not religious, but thank you.

'I have been speaking to one of your friends at the school gates and she agrees with me that we feel that you need to make more of an effort.'

My thoughts: I thought I was making an effort! If only she knew that I make an effort to get out of bed every morning. I make an effort to get dressed. I make an effort to iron my husband's shirt for work. I MAKE AN EFFORT TO STAY ALIVE.

'The mind works in mysterious ways.'

My thoughts: It is a mystery, that's for sure.

An example of one telephone conversation:

'I had to ring because she told me you were really ill.'

'Yes, I have severe depression and anxiety.'

'Oh, thank goodness. I thought it was something serious. I am so relieved.'

My thoughts: If only you could see into my brain, you would realise just how serious it is.

'What do you think the trigger was?'

<u>My thoughts:</u> I have no more idea than you do.

'What do *you* think has caused this?'

<u>My thoughts:</u> I have no more idea than you do.

An example of a conversation:

'Of course you will be working again at some point. We want to have some money.'

I have taken a sleeping pill but wonder how I will get to sleep now. I say, 'Maybe in January I can start thinking about work.'

'I don't think it will be that soon,' he tells me. I feel both relieved and sad.

An example of a conversation:

The doctor says, *'You seem a bit better.'*

'That is what my husband says,' I tell her. But I think to myself that I still feel hopeless. I still sit in the lounge with the TV off staring out of the window. Without my writing, I would be completely unanchored. I am struggling to go out and I certainly can't drive. Mine is not a life at the moment, it is a mere existence.

I tell her, 'I still don't see any point to anything.'

'I think we should increase the Sertraline to 100mg.' She says this as if she is sprinkling the air with stardust, like it is something wonderful.

CHAPTER 12

Well, you look alright to me

"John does not know really how much I suffer. He knows there is no reason to suffer, so this satisfies him."
- Charlotte Perkins Gilman, *The Yellow Wallpaper*

The weekend arrives and my husband is dressed in his black Lycra again, ready for his hours on the bike. He looks very lithe and quite handsome, I guess. Worryingly, I feel nothing.

He asked me last night, 'Will I have sex again?' I replied, 'Of course you will. It might just not be with me.' Has the switch in my brain flicked to off? Am I now going to continually hurt the people that are only trying to love and support me? It would appear so.

Today, the bush from next door's garden has blown over in the wind and it is now obscuring the kitchen window. It is intrusive and blocks the view and the light into the kitchen. I think it is a lobelia, but I am not completely sure.

I often stand at the sink, looking out to admire my little garden. Undoubtedly it is a room with a view. Even in winter the garden looks pleasant. Foliage of different shades of green and some russet reds fill the borders. Little blue pots peep out from behind the shrubs, like children playing hide and seek. When everything is in bloom, the garden goes from a blank canvas to a picture filled with colour: pink, blue, white, lilac and yellow bursting out from every direction. After it has rained, the droplets on the leaves glisten like tiny diamonds and add another lovely dimension.

But for now my view is obscured so I tell my husband I need him to get the shears from the grow house and cut the lobelia back. For some reason, I even make the cutting action with my hands.

He looks at me quizzically. 'But it's next door's,' he says. He goes outside anyway and tries to push back the bush but fails. I am frantically mouthing at him through the window to get the shears while making wild cutting actions with my hands again. It's all a bit dramatic, I know.

He comes back in and then goes outside again. He goes next door to see if the neighbours are in but they aren't. He tries the side gate but it is locked. I think to myself that you can't go onto someone else's property. 'I'll have to leave it for now,' he tells me. I imagine he's anxious to get out on his bike and away from his crazy wife. In my head the voice is screaming, *But what about my view!*

I am left with green leaves and thick branches pressing up against the glass. It is as if they are trying to get in. I can see the veins in the leaves; they are saying to me, 'See, we have veins. We are alive. We are going to break through the glass and tie ourselves firmly around your neck, and pull tighter and tighter until you pass out.'

As I stand transfixed by the veins, I am reminded of a book I once read called *The Yellow Wallpaper* by Charlotte Perkins Gilman. It is a short story about a woman who is suffering from depression. Due to her current mental indisposition, she is taken to a country retreat for three months by her physician husband, John. The woman knows he doesn't believe she is ill because, to him, she looks perfectly fine. There are no visible bleeding wounds or swollen parts of the body.

It is the hidden cloak of mental illness that makes it so cruel because, not only does it make you feel isolated and paranoid, it also plays tricks on your mind. You start to question whether you really are ill.

The woman in the book is locked in a room with bars on the windows and yellow wallpaper. Her husband feels that this is the best course of treatment for her. Immediately she loathes the wallpaper and, due to her being alone for long periods, she becomes fixated on it. She starts to analyse the pattern's curves and twists and feels that she has to decipher them. The feeling starts to overwhelm her and becomes her sole purpose. Although she begins to improve outwardly (which comforts her husband), she is convinced she can see a woman in the wallpaper on all fours who is 'creeping'. Eventually, the woman rips off the paper with the help of this imaginary woman. At the end of the story, the husband enters the room and sees her 'creeping around on all fours' and he faints. To him, it appears that she has gone quite mad.

Gilman suffered from depression, and her treatment from the doctor was the famous 'rest cure'. She tried this for a while; not surprisingly, it didn't help at all. Thankfully the treatment for depression has evolved significantly since then, and the idea of locking a suffering person away in solitary confinement would be considered a form of abuse. I mean, that would cause even the sanest person to go slightly mad.

A few days later, my neighbour is at the front door. He tells me, 'I have just come round to sort out the lavatera.' That's what it's called; I knew it began with a L! 'My wife said it was leaning over the fence quite badly.'

I only have the front door open slightly and I really want him to go away. No one can come into this house.

He gives me an odd look and says, 'I will need to come through and try and push it back.'

I have no choice; I'll have to let him in. I make an excuse that I need to go to the toilet and I run upstairs. I sit on my bed and wish that he would hurry up and leave. After what seems like ages, he shouts to me that he has finished. There is a brief pause and then he tells me he's leaving.

As soon as I hear him close the door, I venture downstairs. He has cut it down completely; I have light in my kitchen again and the green leaves with the strong veins are no longer clawing at the window. The relief I feel is enormous.

A bit later, the postman delivers a letter. It's from the Link counselling service with the date and time of my initial assessment. It says that following this, I will most likely be put on a waiting list until a counsellor can see me. This might take up to three months, possibly longer.

I feel my heart sink with disappointment; I thought this was going to be the start of something. I become breathless and have to concentrate on taking deep breaths in and out. In three months' time, my brain will be a malformed, distorted, stinking mass.

My husband told me the other night that a colleague at work who has a bad knee is being seen straight away. It seems all wrong somehow, but I guess his problem can be seen on an X-ray.

CHAPTER 13

The assessments

"You were testing me "it's my job to test you." I thought it was your job to teach me. That's not the same thing."
- Leigh Bardugo, *Ninth House*

Last night, as we were watching TV, my husband said to me, 'I've been alright to you, haven't I?' It came out of the blue; I guess he is trying to make sense of it all and feels guilty in some way.

I tell him automatically, 'You've been a kind, loving and supportive husband.' That's surely what he needs to hear, isn't it?

I have to ring the cognitive behaviour therapy service today. My doctor gave me a leaflet to read about it, but of course I haven't. I go into the kitchen where it sits on the top of the microwave. It tells me that COGNITIVE refers to our thoughts, memories and images, and the meanings we give to our experiences. BEHAVIOUR refers to everything we do. This includes what we say, how we solve problems, how we act and how we avoid.

When we have emotional problems, such as depression or anxiety, our thinking patterns tend to change and we focus more on the negative side of things.

I know I have to make that phone call because it is a step forward, but ringing them is admitting out loud to the world that I have something wrong with me. And it's not a dodgy knee or a tumour, it's a mental health problem. I feel like I need to whisper it, just in case someone hears.

The leaflet tells me that my first appointment will be to assess what support will be best for me. That could be self-help books, self-help group work (I don't think so), or individual therapy (better idea). These will all work to help me find 'techniques and strategies to bring about change'.

I can't make the phone call from the lounge because it is too open; the window is too big and people walking past can look inside. I decide to use the phone upstairs where it is smaller, cosier, warmer and safer.

My hands are shaking and my mouth is drying out as I wait for the line to connect. The lady on the other end of the phone has a nice soothing voice. She begins by asking me questions to confirm my name, date of birth, address, postcode, ethnicity, religious preferences and marital status. She calls me Rebecca, which would usually bother me as I prefer to be called Becky. Today it doesn't matter because it's like she isn't talking about me but someone else.

I have a telephone appointment booked with a therapist for Wednesday 9th December at 10.30am. The session will last thirty minutes. That sounds like an eternity and I wonder how I will fill the time. She tells me that, in the meantime, a questionnaire will be sent out for me to fill in about how I am feeling. The therapist will go through this with me.

As she goes to get the diary to check the appointment, I am left hanging on the other end of the phone. I feel really lost and look around anxiously. Relief sweeps through my body when her soothing voice returns. The appointment is booked; now all I need to do is to make sure I answer the phone on that day.

I am exhausted. I will have to lie down and close my eyes. I am upstairs anyway, so that will be easy.

A couple of days later I receive the questionnaire in the post. The form states that people's problems sometimes affect their ability to carry out certain day-to-day tasks. In order for them to rate my problems, I have to look at each section and determine on the scale provided how much my problems impair my ability to carry out the activity. The scale ranges from *0: Not at all* to *8: Severely*.

Home management: i.e. cleaning, looking after home/children.

I am definitely NOT doing any cleaning, but I am managing to keep the house quite tidy. I am looking after my son, albeit with a lot of help from others, and I can manage to do some washing. My old self would be on the go constantly, with endless lists of jobs to complete, working hard all the time. I score myself a 4.

Social/leisure activities:

I have gone from being very sociable, with a calendar full of activities and get togethers, to a virtual recluse. All of those outings have been cancelled. I score myself an 8.

Private leisure activities:

I have always enjoyed gardening, walking and running, but now I don't leave the house. I have no desire to start a new book – that would be impossible – but I can revisit my old texts as they are familiar to me. I score myself a 6.

Family and relationships:

I have a lovely family and some wonderful friends, but the only person who gives me any real purpose at the moment is my son. I score myself a 5.

My total score is 31. I guess what that means will be revealed at my appointment.

In the next section, the scores are between *0: Not at all* and *3 Nearly every day*.

Over the past 2 weeks have you been bothered by any of the following problems: Feeling down, depressed or hopeless?

I'm not sure that the person compiling the questionnaire received the memo! I score myself 2 (more than half the days).

Trouble falling or staying asleep or sleeping too much?

As I have been taking medication, it's difficult to gauge how I should answer this. I score myself 1 (several days).

Feeling tired or having little energy.

In my present state, I am extremely lethargic. I score myself a 2.

Moving or speaking so slowly that other people could have noticed, or the opposite: being so fidgety or restless that you have been moving around a lot more than usual.

I'm not speaking to anyone at the moment. My husband is the only person I see regularly, and he often likes to be quiet when he gets home from work. I do think I am speaking more slowly than usual, though. I talk to the cats a lot … maybe they will know? I wouldn't say that I am restless, but I am more apathetic. I spend hours either sitting or lying down doing nothing. I score myself 2 (more than half the days).

Have you had thoughts that you would be better off dead or of hurting yourself in some way?

If I am completely honest, there have been occasions where I have felt this and had the scissors in my hand again, but I didn't cut. I score myself 1 (several days)

There are more questions to complete regarding my handling of social situations and whether I avoid them. At the moment I struggle with collecting the rubbish bins; as for social situations, I am avoiding them totally. The thought makes my jaw tingle. Eventually I complete the form and feel relieved because it is one less thing to worry about. I just need to get my husband to post it.

I feel calmer now, so I think I may tackle the bins after all. I am afraid of someone seeing me or noticing that I don't position them in the correct location. The rain looks like it is coming so if I don't do it now, I won't ever do it.

Reader, I did it! Seventy-four steps in total there and back. I had to walk around my car as it was parked too close to the bins – I cursed that, but I did it!

It felt like it took an eternity and life seemed to go in slow motion. Everything around me seemed so wide and open. The ground seemed to shift underneath me, and I felt like I was going to be swept up into the vastness of my surroundings. When I heard the Royal Mail van coming down the road, I had to run into the house and lock the door. My hands were shaking so much, and my heart felt like it was going to burst out of my chest. Now I am back in the house and I am safe.

My phone pings and I read a text from my best friend, Becky. She has texted me very day since this all started.

How are you doing? she asks.

I tell her about the rubbish, and she tells me well done, take it slowly. I tell her I thought I might walk to the postbox to post a birthday card, then I realised that I couldn't do that today. But I am so proud that I took out the rubbish.

Small steps, she texts.

A few days later...

The telephone appointment:

The first question from the lady on the phone from the cognitive behavioural therapy service is, 'Have you had any thoughts of suicide or harming yourself in any way?'

I can imagine her sitting at her desk reading the questions methodically from a sheet. *There's nothing like starting with a bang!* I think to myself. I seem to be getting asked that a lot lately. I think about the scissors, but I didn't do myself any real damage so I answer no.

' Have you ever taken an overdose of medication?' Isn't that similar to what she's just asked me? Or is taking an overdose of medication not considered hurting yourself? Maybe it could mean cod liver oil tablets. But now I'm just being ridiculous. I tell her no.

' Have you ever had any other episodes of depression?' Her voice sounds mechanical.

I tell her that I had one episode when my dad died back in 1997. I was on a short course of fluoxetine that made me talk incessantly, have an abundance of energy and not sleep. Then I feel really guilty; how can I be more ill now, when losing my dad was the worst thing in the world?

'Have you ever shown any aggression or had any issues with it in the past?'

I tell her that I am a placid person. I can't remember kicking or throwing anything in anger in my life.

The counsellor goes through the questionnaire that I was sent to try to establish what has led me to be like this now, trying to see what the trigger was or if there was one at all. She asks me about my difficulties in trying to leave the house.

'Just the feeling of openness really,' I say. It sounds so lame. Then I tell her about how I struggle to get to the rubbish bins in and how I struggle walking to the end of the road, and I begin to feel more genuine. I tell her I hate the thought of people seeing me, looking at me. I feel that they are judging me.

'Oh, this is so pathetic being like this,' I suddenly blurt out.

'Why do you say it's pathetic?' she asks in a kindly voice.

'Well, I just am. I am trying to fight it. I don't want to be like this. I want to go out and stop feeling like this. But I just can't,' I say.

She congratulates me on making the initial phone call to book the telephone assessment. 'It seems to me that you want to seek help to get better.'

'Doesn't everyone?' I ask.

She tells me that some clients haven't been out of the house for years. One individual hasn't left their house for nearly twenty years. I feel guilty again, fraudulent, and also I could weep for those people. I just don't know how to process the remorse I feel for them; it is overwhelming.

When I tell her about my journal writing, she says that she is pleased that I'm taking steps to help myself. 'So how do you want to proceed? What help do you think you need?'

I think to myself, *Shouldn't you be telling me this?* I'm still reeling from the information regarding her poor clients inside their houses for years.

Eventually she breaks the heavy silence. 'I think we should address the anxiety first with a one-to-one appointment for some CBT exercises to at least get you functioning a bit better. Then we can address the depression with some counselling sessions, which will be a longer process.'

Because the agoraphobia has only been evident for weeks, rather than months or years, she is hoping that I will benefit from some exercises and techniques. They will send me an appointment for the CBT sessions.

The conversation is at an end. I put down the phone utterly exhausted. I forgot to ask her how long the appointment would take to arrive. I wonder how I am supposed to get to the appointment if I am agoraphobic. It's quite comical, really.

For now, I'll just keep unburdening my thoughts onto the pages of my pink notebook.

CHAPTER 14

Those little moments

"Last night I dreamt I went to Manderley again."
- Daphne Du Maurier, *Rebecca*

My routine was slightly different this morning because my nine-year-old son woke up and declared he had a tummy ache. 'Really?' I say. 'Or do you just not want to go to school.'

He protests as adamantly as he can. 'No, I really do. I do!'

I give him some Calpol and at the same time I take two paracetamol because my head is pounding. My mouth tastes disgusting again. Maybe I really am rotting inside.

My husband is downstairs eating his porridge, and he looks at me hopefully. Nothing has changed, I want to yell at him. Just because I got out of bed on my own this morning, NOTHING

HAS CHANGED! He told me last night that he thinks I am improving but I know I'm not.

My husband forces my son to get dressed. It turns out he hasn't really got tummy ache, but he doesn't understand why I'm not going to work. 'I don't argue with you! I don't tell you you aren't ill! it's not fair!'

He is right in thinking that. None of this is fair.

My head is still pounding despite the paracetamol. Boom! Boom! Boom!

I read a text message from a friend: Writing is good. It is a powerful voice. All paths lead to a destination, however dark. Yours will lead back to life.

It sounds like something from a self-help book, but I know she means well.

The house is so quiet now apart from the ticking of the clock. Every second that passes is a moment lost forever. The only sounds are my pen scribbling in my notebook and Sheamus licking his fur.

I feel so lightheaded and groggy. It's the sleeping tablets. Maybe I should try half a tablet tonight. Will I have the strength to do that, I wonder?

Last night I emptied my bedside table drawer, which was full of work stuff. I threw it all into a black dustbin bag and chucked it out of sight in the corner of my wardrobe. I filled the drawer with books, a thesaurus and my writing implements. Now it looks just as it should be. It is perfect.

All I want to do is go back to bed, but I must write some pages in my notebook because I feel it is helping.

My best friend is visiting me this afternoon and I know she will hold my hand through this. When we first met each other, we were both seven years old. Her family had relocated from London to Bexhill-on-Sea. I recall the exact day: I was at school and the teacher told me I had to look after her as we both had the same name, Rebecca.

I remember being transfixed by her hair; it was pure white, like beautiful spun silk. Mine was a mousey-brown colour. I don't think I'd seen anything like it before. And I remember she was wearing a dress; I can't recall the colour or design of it, but I know I thought she looked really pretty. That is my first memory of her.

Since that first day we have looked after each other. She has done more of the looking after, but I hope I have done my part as well. I guess I must have because she is arriving this afternoon.

Today it only seems right that I pick up the novel *Rebecca* by Daphne Du Maurier as we are both called Rebecca. The book was a gift from my dad on my fourteenth birthday. I don't think he had any idea what it was about and bought it because of the title. I liked the author's name because it sounded so exotic.

I used to carry it around with me all the time. I even took it to school and sometimes would sit on the toilet and get lost in the text. My copy is well worn and some of the pages have been sell-otaped in. My school mates used to tease me and say, 'You're not reading that again, are you? You do know that it's not about you?'

This is a book I have read countless times, and the one book I would try to save if there was ever a fire in my house. I treasure it.

The novel begins with the narrator seeing Manderley in a dream. Nature has obscured the view of the great house; it now lays in ruins which she says is a 'sepulchre of our pain and suffering.' That is the book's magic, the sense of suspense.

At the centre of the story is this ancient crumbling mansion, Manderley, the home of Maxim de Winter. Du Maurier describes the ocean as lying just the other side of the rose garden. From my first reading of the book I felt an instant connection to this because I grew up by the sea. Even as I read the novel now, I long to live in Manderley and stand on its beautiful, manicured lawn. I can imagine breathing in the salty air and listening to the waves crashing on the rocks, letting the atmosphere fill up my senses.

When the narrator first meets Maxim, she is a shy young girl with no confidence. As a somewhat bashful fourteen year old, I identified strongly with the character. They meet in Monte Carlo; he is a widower, seemingly trying to come to terms with his wife Rebecca's death, and the narrator is a travelling companion for the ghastly Mrs Van Hopper. The two of them fall in love and he quickly proposes.

Similarly to Jane Eyre, the second Mrs de Winter has many obstacles to overcome. When Maxim takes her to Manderley, she is eclipsed by Rebecca who lives on beyond the grave in every inch of the house. This inevitably makes her feel anxious, tearful and inadequate. I am the youngest of three girls in my family. When I was growing up, I felt my two older sisters received most of the attention and often overshadowed me, so I can relate to how this character feels.

The housekeeper, Mrs Danvers, plays mind games with Mrs de Winter. She wants her to fail as mistress of Manderley because Mrs Danvers continues to love Rebecca. Shakespeare writes in *Macbeth*, *'something wicked this way comes'*, which reminds me of Mrs Danvers. I remember at fourteen being scared to death of her; if I'm completely truthful, I still am to a certain extent.

The twist in the book is the truth that Maxim never loved Rebecca, who was an evil, manipulative person. He shot her during an argument when she was pregnant with another man's baby, put her body in a boat and sank it. In reality Rebecca wasn't pregnant but dying from a cancer that had ravished her body. When her body is recovered it seems that all will be revealed and Maxim will hang for his crime, but he is saved by her cancer diagnosis as it is believed that it drove her to commit suicide. With the secret they share, and the knowledge that Maxim didn't love Rebecca, the narrator becomes a confident person who can support her husband – although, as she says, 'I suppose it is his dependence on me that has made me bold.'

By the end of the novel, Manderley lies in ashes and the couple live in exile. It is a life that is often dull and monotonous but that doesn't matter; they are free from fear and they learn to appreciate the simplicity of it. The narrator says, *'Happiness is not a possession to be prized, it is a quality of thought, a state of mind.'*

I remember listening to the *Jeremy Vine Show* recently when he was interviewing a Macmillan nurse. He asked her what was the most common regret people had when they knew they were going to die. She said it was that they wished they'd realised that they could have chosen to be happy.

Depression feels like you are in a car and you are heading towards a cliff. You try the brakes but they don't work, and you realise you are going over the edge. All that you can do is hold on tight and hope that somehow you will survive.

Somehow I have to learn that the most incidental things can bring the most joy, like planting a tulip bulb in the garden and watching it grow into an elegant flower. Like the excited feeling I had when picking blackberries all those years ago with my grandma. I need to really appreciate the trees, the garden and birds. I remember my dad saying to me that life is all about the gold nuggets; I need to treasure them and let them fill my mind with brightness.

The following week, my best friend visits me again. I have another doctor's appointment to attend and she takes me. As we sit in the waiting room, we both notice two posters on the wall. One advertises bipolar disorder group meetings at a community centre. Above that, the other poster says, *Are you worried about your memory?* We both laugh because there is me in my present state and her with her episodes of forgetting things. Mostly she will forget a word in a sentence; one time she couldn't remember the word 'chocolate'. She has Alzheimer's in her family.

I tell the doctor about my writing. I say, 'I do it from 8.30am until 1pm every day and then I wait for my son to return from school.'

Although she seems pleased, she looks at me for a while then says, 'Maybe we should increase your antidepressants? The maximum dose is 200mg.'

Later on my friend buys me a prawn sandwich. She tells me it is for us to share and she puts one half on a plate for me. I only ate two crackers and a handful of blueberries before she arrived, so I am hungry. I eat the sandwich and, even though it is the simplest of things, it is rather nice.

Later I go with her to pick my son up from school. I stay in the car where I feel safe whilst she goes down to the school gates to meet him. It is a massive step forward for me and I know I have only managed this because of her. As I sit there and watch her walking back towards the car with her arm round my son, I am so thankful that on her first day of school I was the only girl there who was called Rebecca.

CHAPTER 15

Daydream believer

"To sleep, perchance to dream."
- William Shakespeare, *Hamlet*

Another month has arrived. I feel like I am losing track of the days, so I have to check on my phone. It is the first of December and the time is 8.26am. As the house is empty of human company I will have to say 'White Rabbits' to the cats.

I only took half a sleeping tablet last night, but it still worked. Last night I dreamt not that I went to Manderley but another vivid dream. I am finding out over time that when you are on these medications it is not a dreamless, peaceful sleep you experience.

I read on the internet that dreams are our subconscious thoughts and a continuation of feelings we have had during the day. Here are some of my dream experiences.

Dream number one

I am in the garden of a friend that I knew many years ago. She has a big garden. We are both sitting enjoying the sunshine when two dogs run past with deep, open, oozing wounds. Their blood is pouring onto the concrete path, but my friend doesn't notice anything. Then another dog runs past with an even deeper wound on its side. I ask myself how he is managing to run so fast with such a big wound. It doesn't seem to bother him at all. Again, my friend notices nothing.

Dream number two

My husband and I are driving down a country lane – I think we are on holiday. Suddenly he demands that I get out of the car. I can't believe this, as we are in the middle of nowhere and I have no handbag, no mobile phone, nothing. I tell him that but he doesn't care. 'Get out,' he says. So I do and he drives off. I am alone in the lane. I wander around for a while and eventually I find the hotel where we are staying. I walk down a corridor, past rooms that are full of old people like a nursing home. Then someone (I think it's the nurse) says to me, 'This way. Your husband is in here.' There he is, standing by the window. 'I can't believe you did that,' I say. 'Did what? I have done nothing,' he says. I try to protest but he is adamant that he hasn't done anything.

Dream number three

I am in town having lunch with my friend and I tell her that I will go and get us two teas from the café around the corner. As I start walking, the area gets less familiar; I am passing souvenir shops and amusement arcades. It reminds me of growing up by the seaside. I keep walking for what seems like ages, and the streets become more and more unfamiliar. I think it is so ridiculous that I can't find the café. Suddenly, I am in a room and two men are kicking a puppy. I yell, 'Hey, don't do that!' and think how brave I am – they could hit me, or worse. But they don't, so I grab the puppy and run. He starts to whimper and I realise he must be hungry. A lady passes me and I ask, 'What shall I give him to eat?' She says, 'Oh for goodness' sake! Just give him some dry biscuits.' I tell her I don't know what to do, but she ignores me and walks on. I look down at the puppy and he is getting smaller and smaller. I start crying, wishing someone would help me.

My thoughts during the day are of feeling lost and alone. I often wonder what will happen to me. I constantly worry about how people see me; I think they either don't care, or don't understand what I am going through. I would say my dreams are pretty accurate.

CHAPTER 16

Love is all around

"I love you to the moon and back."
- Sam McBratney, *Guess How Much I Love You*

I find it hard to open my eyes this morning.

My husband asks, 'Are you getting up this morning?'

'It's 7.30am. I'll get up at 7.45am,' I say.

'No, you need to get up now because I've got to go to the shop to get milk and cat food, and you need to sort out Archie for school.'

I get up, but my limbs feel heavy and my head is swimming. I stumble downstairs and start to make my husband a sandwich to take to work. With me not working, he can't be buying lunch every day. Two slices of granary bread. Sliced chorizo and cheese. It's an effort but I manage it.

'Don't use that chorizo, it's seen better days,' my husband says.

'I don't know why I bother,' I mutter.

'I don't mean it like that. Look, there's a bowl of tuna mayonnaise in the fridge that I've made up. You don't want me to get sick, do you?' He winks at me. I was always a sucker for his winks.

'Fine. Sorry,' I say, pondering the thought of him being sick.

'I need you to iron me a shirt as well,' he says.

I feel like the jobs are piling up. I haven't put out the cat food yet or emptied the dishwasher. Then my son appears half dressed for school, no socks or jumper on. He is playing some game on his iPad. I make him a crumpet and then go to iron the shirt.

'I'm not hungry,' he says.

'What about porridge?' I ask.

'Okay.'

The first attempt I add too much milk, so I have to bin it. The second bowl is okay and he eats half. I eat the crumpet, quickly stuffing it into my mouth. At least I've had breakfast, so that's one less job to worry about. I manage to iron the shirt.

My husband appears. Sensing my stress, he rests his hand on my shoulder. 'It's alright, there is no rush.'

'But I'm behind with my jobs. I'm not even dressed, and I have to be on the sofa by 8.30am, ready to write.' My breath catches in my throat.

He gives me a strange look then a quick kiss goodbye.

My son appears, now appropriately dressed. I give him a kiss goodbye. His cheek is so soft.

I make it on time, 8.28am.

My son means everything to me. How do people go through something like this without children? Children give you a reason to get out of bed in the morning and try to function because they need you to. The love you feel for them comes before anything else in life. One thing that I have done since my son was a toddler is to read him a bedtime story then tuck him up in his bed, surrounded by his stuffed animals. He tells me he likes me doing that as his dad doesn't do it properly. I tuck him in properly, making him all snug under the duvet, but apparently my husband just throws the duvet over him and says 'Night night!' before hurrying out of the room.

I've done this since he was little. I give him a kiss on both cheeks to see which one is the softest. Sometimes it is easy and straight away I say, 'That one!' and point at the appropriate cheek. Last night, when I was tucking him, I couldn't decide. 'Not sure,' I said.

He promptly checked himself by prodding each cheek. 'This one,' he said, pointing at the right one. 'It's bouncier.'

'Yes, I think you are right,' I said. It pulled at my heartstrings the way he looked up at me with his big blue eyes.

He doesn't believe I am sick. He says I'm faking it so I don't have to go to work. He doesn't understand because I am up and around, not being sick or complaining that I have a headache or tummy ache. He wouldn't want to know what is going on in my cerebrum. It's aching so much that I think parts of it have died. I tell him that when I am better I will be able take him to school again and pick him up.

'Yay!' is his response. 'And you won't have any nights away when you are working?' he asks.

Before all of this, I worked as a medical rep so nights away were part of my job. I tell him that I won't. I know that I can't go back to that world because I won't follow the same paths. I have to do something different with my life. Hopefully I will work again, although at the moment that feels a long way off. I just have to hope that I will get there. To see more of my son, though, will be wonderful.

When he was born, he was eleven days late. His lungs were full of meconium, which he had inhaled due to being in severe distress. He was rushed to Leicester Glenfield Hospital and received treatment from an ECMO machine. This stands for extracorporeal membrane oxygenation and it mimics the work of the heart and lungs, oxygenating the blood so that those organs can rest. Meanwhile his lungs were being cleaned.

When he was in his little transporter with tubes everywhere, waiting to be transferred, I felt like someone was ripping my heart from my chest. I'd had a Caesarean section, so I had to stay in hospital. When I was eventually reunited with him at Leicester Hospital, my husband and I stayed in a relatives' room. I remember I had to use a breast pump so that my son could be given some milk. When I used it on one breast, milk would pour out of the other while the tears flowed down my cheeks. My husband wheeled me round the hospital in a wheelchair as massive clots came out of me and milk soaked through my tops.

The midwife told me that I'd been so lucky to not have lost my son. 'You have a guardian angel on both of your shoulders,' she told me, and I know it is my dad.

My son is nine years old now and has grown up tall and strong. A tiny scar on his neck is the only visible mark from his ordeal. He is kind and sweet natured, and I am very proud of him. I hope I can guide him onto the right path in life, and that he has some good luck as well.

Today, because I have been writing about my son, my head feels clearer. It's rather like suddenly being able to see the bottom of the sea because all the muddy water has finally disappeared.

CHAPTER 17

It's all in the genes?

"I am drowning, my dear, in seas of fire."
- Virginia Woolf, *To the Lighthouse*

My husband and I joked last night that me sitting at home writing my 'musings', as he describes them, likens me to Virginia Woolf.

I'm in my usual place, sitting writing in the lounge, looking out at the trees. I start searching the internet for more information on Virginia. I learn that her mental illness is described as a 'manic depressive illness', more commonly known as bipolar disorder. The NHS website describes it as: 'a condition that affects your mood which can swing from one extreme to another.' There are periods or episodes of depression where you feel very low and lethargic and have thoughts of suicide. Then there is a manic phase where you feel very high and overactive, not wanting to eat or sleep. Talking quickly and becoming annoyed easily are common characteristics of this phase.

Virginia was a victim of her time when there was a lack of support and understanding of mental health. The therapy she received really only consisted of rest. Near the end of her life she feared she had lost her ability to write, which was too much for her to bear. Some say that the treatment she received from her husband, Leonard, encouraged her ill health; others say he gave her immense support so she was able to live as long as she did. This is affirmed in her last note to him: *Dearest, I feel certain that I am going mad again. And I shan't recover this time. You have given me the greatest possible happiness. You have been in every way all that anyone could be.*

On her third attempt at suicide she succeeded. She drowned herself in the River Ouse at the age of fifty-nine.

Lots of causes are cited for her condition and eventual downfall. Her mother died, her father remarried and she was abused by her half-brothers. Stella, her half-sister who she was very close to, died, and then her father died.

There was a history of mental illness in Virginia's family. Her grandfather and her half-sister Laura both suffered, and Laura was placed in an asylum.

Both she and Virginia faced their own battles. If this illness was in the genes, maybe Virginia was always going to be susceptible. Maybe the abuse and grief she experienced triggered it. Perhaps life triggered it.

That gets me thinking about the question I keep getting asked: What do you think has caused your depression? As Stephen Fry has said, there may be no specific reason. Anyone can get depression, whether they are a queen or a pauper. But I have knowledge of mental illness in my family, so the genetic link always comes to mind.

As far as I'm aware, my parents had no history of mental illness although my mum is, let's say, quirky. But when I turn to my grandparents, it gets interesting. My father's mum, who my sisters and I called Nana, was a small, thin lady with long grey hair that lay sparsely on her shoulders. She had long bony fingers and light-blue eyes. I remember her face being expressionless, a blank. It was neither a kind nor an unkind face. I used to ask my mum, 'Is the witch coming to see us today?' Nana was like the witch that I had nightmares about who was hiding in the wardrobe next to my bed – except Nana's face wasn't green.

I remember Nana brought me a cot that I desperately wanted for one of my dolls, and I was really confused because I believed she didn't love me. One day she turned up at the house and threatened my mum. She stood in the doorway, her thin hair hanging around her thin face, holding a large silver knife. I remember Mum telling me and my sisters to go upstairs into the bedroom and lock the door. Nana didn't attack my mum, just abused her verbally. That was the final straw. We never saw her again because my mum and dad broke contact with her.

When I was older, Mum told me that Nana was schizophrenic. I looked on the NHS website about her condition; of course, there is plenty of information.

Schizophrenia is a long-term mental health condition that causes a range of different psychological symptoms including hallucinations, delusions, and changes in behaviour. Doctors often describe it as a psychotic illness. This means that sometimes a person may not self-help distinguish their own thoughts and ideas from reality.

The symptoms of schizophrenia are either positive or negative.

Positive symptoms represent a change in behaviour or thoughts, such as hallucinations or delusions.

Negative symptoms represent a withdrawal or lack of function that you would expect to see in a healthy person. For example, people with schizophrenia often appear expressionless, flat and apathetic.

I have mentioned that Nana's face was often blank. I don't remember her ever laughing or crying.

What she went through with her illness must have been awful, but my poor dad suffered. He was an only child who never knew his real father who had left when Dad was a baby. Because his mum couldn't look after him properly, Dad was put in children's homes. He hated them and used to run away. He died aged sixty from lymphoma. I believe his mother lived well into her nineties. It's funny how life goes.

Although depression is known to run in families, the research into genetics is in the early stages. I found a quote on the internet by Mehmet Oz, which I thought summed it up rather well:

Think of it this way, your genes load the gun but it's your behaviour and environment that pull the trigger.

I think that I was always susceptible to this disease; it was always hiding away waiting to pounce. One day it did, when my life and I brought it out of the shadows into the light, bringing its demons with it.

CHAPTER 18

It must be nature, then?

"There it was before her – life ... oddly enough she must admit that she felt this thing that she called life terrible, hostile and quick to pounce on you if you gave it a chance."
- Virginia Woolf, *To the Lighthouse*

I get up with a struggle at 7am. I took half a sleeping tablet last night. I was in bed at 9.30pm, wide awake, waiting for it to work, thinking I would never get to sleep. Then suddenly it was 5.30am and the cats were crying to be let out.

When I buttered my toast this morning, I had to be very sparing with the margarine as the new one in the fridge needed to be thrown away; Sheamus had got onto the kitchen work surface and licked it. All my son and I could hear from upstairs was my husband shouting, 'You are a fat ginger pig!' My son clapped his hands and we both laughed. The little devil had taken his chance when everyone's back was turned to grab himself a little treat. Good for him!

The house is now quiet, apart from the washing in the machine going round. I can still manage to do that. The cats have licked their bowls clean. I gave them some sardines earlier, another treat for Sheamus. I like to spoil them; it makes me feel good.

The dustmen are here as it's recycling day. My husband put the bins out this morning and I didn't even have to ask him. When I look at the dustmen outside my lounge window they look so happy, laughing and joking with each other. Maybe the simplicity of carrying out their tasks gives them joy. They enjoy their simple life, just like Mrs de Winter.

Yesterday my husband brought me some lovely roses . Whenever I pass a rose, I always smell it; the smell of a rose is like a little drop of happiness. I know it will remind me of my grandma. She grew beautiful yellow, white and pink roses. She was an incredibly strong lady, both physically and mentally. Together with always working hard and keeping busy, she lived alone because her husband (my maternal grandfather) died from cancer in his forties. She didn't meet anyone else to share her life with. She managed on very little money.

I remember at my grandma's there was an outdoor toilet and a potty under the bed if we needed to pee in the night. When I was little I never used the potty because that was where the goblins and witches lived. By the time I was older and my nightmares had gone, Grandma had installed a fully-fitted bathroom.

One day some years later, the switch in her brain flicked to off and she sort of gave up. She lived with my parents for a while. I remember coming back from work and she'd be sitting in the chair, staring at the wall. She would sit like that for hours. Eventually my parents felt she would cope better in a residential home. She enjoyed it, and I think it was a nice place. She used to sit in the lounge talking to the other residents and it did her good.

Although she lived there for five years, she never once took a step outside not even to go into the garden, despite loving gardening throughout her life. She died in 2002 after a stroke and her ashes are scattered over the fields that she loved to walk through with her many different dogs.

Life ... it has a lot to answer for. There are many things that I have had to face in my life that I could cite as reasons for my present predicament. Heartbreak, the death of my dad, my mum having cancer, heartbreak again. I recall that old saying that what doesn't break you makes you stronger, but I don't know whether that's entirely true. All of the hardships in life chip away at your mind until there is not enough left for it to function properly. I think that's why I am always drawn to books where the characters have to struggle and overcome.

Today I open the only book by Virginia Woolf that I have read, *To the Lighthouse*. The reason I love this book so much is because it shows the particulars of life with painful clarity. The story centres around a close-knit family, the Ramsays, and their visits to the Isle of Skye between 1910 and 1920. The death of Mrs Ramsay, and how the family deal with her passing, is central to the story. The book highlights how the characters see each other, how they interact with each other and how this affects them individually. That is its triumph, because the web of human emotion is so deeply woven throughout the book.

A trip is planned to the lighthouse prior to Mrs Ramsey's death, but it never happens. The remaining members of the family return ten years later and attempt it again. The lighthouse is a symbol of hope and constancy, and the characters are always trying to move towards it to gain some sort of validation and completeness within their lives.

The sea is so choppy that it appears unlikely they will succeed. Lily Briscoe, a painter and a close family friend who often holidays with them, is on land painting. She is trying to finish a painting that she had started years before. She watches the boat with Mr Ramsay and two of his children, James and Cam, attempting to reach the lighthouse and thinks that it looks impossible. As she stands there, she starts to think about Mrs Ramsay and is overcome with emptiness and the realisation that nothing lasts forever. Even the painting she is attempting to finish will be discarded.

On the boat, the fisherman's son cuts a piece out of the side of a fish for bait and throws the mutilated, live body back into the sea. When I read this bit, it always makes me think of the cruelty of life but also the possibility of surviving whatever pain life can bring. At the same time, the image of the poor, discarded fish floundering around the ocean trying to survive makes me think you may survive – but at what cost? How fulfilling can your life be following a traumatic event such as having part of your body removed, or a mental breakdown. I imagine the fish in the sea didn't live long. Or perhaps it did, its wounds healed, and the other fish sympathised and understood why it couldn't swim properly. His wound was visible, not the invisible wound of mental illness.

Lily is still crying on the shore, but eventually her intense pain subsides and she sees, much to her relief, that the boat has reached the lighthouse. Even though she is exhausted by her emotions, she manages to finish her painting. She can finally see what is needed through the blurred lines and the greens and blues;

she draws a line in the centre and realises that the painting is finally complete.

As a reader, I always interpret the ending as the characters reaching a point of peace and acceptance with themselves and life. For the depressed person, believing that point can ever be reached is difficult but even attempting to attain it can only be viewed as a positive step, and for that we should be proud of ourselves.

I notice that my neighbour has kindly taken in the dustbin for me, so at least for today I don't have to worry about steps.

CHAPTER 19

Love again

"If you live to be a hundred, I want to live to be a hundred minus one day, so I never have to live without you."
- A. Milne, *Winnie the Pooh*

The trees look tired this morning, nearly at the end of their annual cycle of growth. They follow the same pattern. Someone texted to advise me not to repeat life's patterns; I can understand that, but the natural cycle is reassuring in its constancy.

I love trees; they are therapeutic to watch. Christmas will soon be here and this one will be tough. As Joni Mitchell sang, 'It's coming on Christmas, they're cutting down trees … oh I wish I had a river I could skate away on.' I would like that, to disappear until it was all over.

My husband is working for a few hours this morning, so it is just me and my son. We make our usual weekend treat of pancakes. I am exhausted after putting flour and an egg into a bowl and mixing it. Adding the milk seems to take all of my concentration and strength. I spill a lot of the milk on the work surface and some of the egg shell falls into the mixture. I remember my grandma using the same ingredients when she made Yorkshire puddings; I loved watching how much effort she put into stirring the spoon around the big brown bowl. The puddings were so light and fluffy that they melted in your mouth.

Earlier on, when I was looking through some paperwork, I found a photo book that my best friend had given to me for my fortieth birthday. It contains pictures of the two of us at different points in our lives. One is of us on the carnival float in Bexhill-on-Sea when we about seven. I look ridiculous with a red-and-white garland round my neck and a silver crown on my head. My mum always made me do the carnivals and I hated it.

There is another sweet photo of us with our dogs. My friend owned a long-haired Corgi called Muffin, and I had a Boxer dog called Henrietta, or Henny, as I called her. My mum named her; in fact, her full name was Henrietta Pearl Doris Marsden. See what I mean about quirky?

The really humorous thing in the book is the note my friend reprinted that I wrote for her when I was about fourteen. It shows how immature I was, even at that age, but it is so funny; reading it now fills me with sadness but makes me smile.

When I get my first book published, I will leave you a copy and sign it inside. If by some remote chance that I don't get it published then here is my autograph to be going on with. You never know, it could be worth a lot of money in a few years. People could be breaking your door down to get the autograph and pay you loads of money for it. So in a way I am helping you to become a millionaire. Cool, eh? Well, if you are ever hard up for a bob or two then you know where to go – not to me! Luv your dearest pal. Then I signed it and dated it.

I never believed that I could write a book; I wrote this note just to try and be funny. '*Believe in yourself and all that you are. Know that there is something inside you greater than any obstacle,*' is another quote that I love by Christian D. Larson.

When I was twenty-five, I completed a writing for publication course at night school. The tutor was German and quite eccentric. She had a passion for belly dancing and wrote many articles about it. She turned up to one class in her costume and did a belly dance for us, and I remember thinking at the time that it was very odd.

As I progressed through the course, I wrote some articles which were published. One was about my working holiday in Australia; I spent a year there when I was twenty-three, and nursed and travelled. The other article was an interview with my friend Julie, who had just come back from a working holiday in America. The third one was for a lifestyle magazine, where I travelled to London to interview a friend who was an opera singer and had landed a role in Cosi fan Tutte.

I absolutely loved the process of interviewing and writing up the articles. Seeing my work in print was so exciting, and I remember everyone in the class clapping at my small successes. I badgered my poor dad to buy an answer machine so I wouldn't miss any publishers who rang me.

I remember I travelled to an animal sanctuary where the owner had agreed to an interview. I thought I had produced a wonderful piece of work, which I called *Sylvia's Haven*, but it didn't get published and then I sort of gave up. I should have persevered but, as always, I struggled with believing in myself. My friend has kept that note all these years and cherished it. Other people believe in me; I just have to learn to start believing in myself.

My son has finished writing his letter to Santa. It's in the envelope addressed with the postcode on it, which we had to Google. When we were addressing the envelope, he asked me if Santa is real. He must have heard some rumours at school. 'I mean, I like the idea of flying reindeers – but really?' he says.

I can't stop the magic yet. He might be almost ten, but I want him to hang onto the innocence of childhood a little bit longer. 'Of course he is real. Don't think about it too much. Don't question it, just believe,' I say.

'But look, you are smiling,' he says.

'Honestly, Santa exists and he always will, as long as you believe. I certainly do.' I remembered a Ronald Dahl quote: 'those who don't believe in magic will never find it.'

He seems satisfied with this. I have an aim to try and post this letter later with him, a small step forward.

My phone rings. It is a text from my best friend who is in London today doing some Christmas shopping.

Do you want me to get you anything?

A new cerebrum? I text back.

What colour?

Pink.

I will see what I can do.

Later she texts to tell me that she couldn't find what I wanted because they weren't as good as the one I already have. Nowhere near.

I think that I'd better try and walk to the postbox, then.

In the end I don't have to walk as far as the postbox as my son runs ahead to post his letter. He is so excited. I am relieved I only have to walk to the end of the road. I am holding my husband's hand so tightly and leaning on him for support. There are a few people on their way to church; a man passes by with his dog and says hello.

I keep my head down. I am wearing a hat and a muffler round my neck, so most of my face is covered. I feel protected, but I still feel incredibly vulnerable and exposed. It is like the whole world is looking at me and judging me – there is the crazy lady who can hardly stand up. My husband asks me if I am okay and tells me to breathe in and out slowly.

The outside feels so open and endless. It feels wrong somehow to put one foot in front of the other. 'Just keep walking,' I tell myself, 'and you will soon be back home safe.'

Somehow I manage to get back in one piece. The house was only out of sight for a few minutes, but when I see it again the relief is enormous. Once inside, I have to sit down, take deep breaths and wait for my heart to slow down.

I don't know how I feel about my achievement. I thought I would feel better, elated, but I just feel worn out and subdued.

We watch a bit of TV to pass the time and shift the focus away from my present state. Sheamus is curled up asleep by my feet looking so sweet. The house is warm, cosy and harmless. I am back within my safety net and all is good for a while.

CHAPTER 20

Running, me?

"The distance is nothing when one has a motive."
- Jane Austen, *Pride and Prejudice*

I'm thinking about exercise today. The doctors keep telling me to go outside for a walk as exercise is good for depression. If only I could go out and enjoy a walk along the canal. I visualise myself doing it and then I feel panic. Hopefully some day soon I will be able to.

I always enjoyed sports at school – netball, hockey, tennis, badminton, even gymnastics. I would have a go at most things and was always a keen participant of sports day. In my adult years I started running. The first thing I trained for was the London Marathon when I was twenty-six. The aim was to raise money for cancer research as I had just lost my dad to that awful disease. Afterwards I carried on running on and off until recently. I've taken part in half-marathons, 10kms runs and 5kms runs, all of which I enjoyed because of the challenge and the lovely feeling it gave me to achieve something..

In terms of running, the most common thinking is that it makes you feel good because it releases endorphins. But after looking on the internet, it seems that the runners' 'high' is not just down to endorphins. The euphoric feeling could, in fact, be due also to endocannabinoids, biochemical substances similar to cannabis but produced naturally by the body. Considering that I am a trained nurse, it's surprising I have never heard of them.

There have been loads of studies that show how exercise improves mood. I hope that the antidepressants will kick-start me into some sort of action. For me, running has always been something I return to even when I don't do it for a while. I think it's addictive; For me, it is a fine line between pleasure and pain. I always find it hard and that is the challenge, but I love the feeling I have afterwards that I have achieved something meaningful. I feel like I am in control because I can set the pace and I don't have to chase a ball or wait for it to land. That sense of control is important, especially when other parts of my life feel like they are falling apart.

It says on the internet that, although regular exercise isn't a cure, it can help with increasing your mood to a point where your depression could be managed. My lovely friend the hippocampus has also been found to be of higher volume in the brains of people taking regular exercise.

If you exercise regularly, you've got more reason to get a big head about your efforts: physical activity increases the size of your brain.

In a new review of the evidence conducted by researchers in Australia, the volume of the left side of the hippocampus was reliably bigger among adults who underwent an aerobic exercise intervention. The hippocampus is critical for the formation of new memories, because its involved in transferring information from short term memory to long term memory. When older adults suffer from a deteriorating hippocampus, it often results in memory loss and disorientation. This review suggests that aerobic exercise could prevent some of the problems that comes with normal ageing, as well as dementia.

www.cambridgebrainsciences.com

It is a sunny day today. I watch the little birds hopping about on the bare twigs, pecking for imaginary berries. I think they are chaffinches but I'm not sure.

It would be good to be able to go outside and feel the crisp, clear, winter's day on my cheeks. To walk along the canal, waving to people on passing boats, watch the ducks and swans glide across the water. I imagine the swans with their legs paddling ferociously under the water feeling exhausted but hiding it with their serenity. I wonder if they feel like giving up sometimes.

My husband tells me he has the day off on Friday, so I don't have to be alone. He will try to take me out somewhere. Maybe a walk along the canal? Maybe I could do it with him supporting me? I like to think I could.

CHAPTER 21

Don't look back in anger

"What's done is done and cannot be undone."
- William Shakespeare, *Macbeth*

There are three hours until my son comes back from school. I spent the morning scribbling in between a lot of time staring out at the trees. They are becoming my friends and I'm sure it won't be long before I start naming them.

I feel a bit better today, a bit brighter somehow. Maybe the medication is starting to work. I think I'm starting to understand how things might happen:

1. The medication will help me get off the sofa and start living.

2. The counselling (when it starts) will help me learn coping mechanisms.

3. The journaling/reading will help me learn about myself.

4. The love of family/friends will help me forget myself.

As I read what I have just written, I realise that I do have a bit of a sense of humour left. Today, instead of going to lie on the bed as I usually do, I decide to read a bit of *Macbeth*. I studied the play for my English Literature O' Level and have loved it ever since, mostly because of Lady Macbeth and all her many flaws.

My English teacher at high school was called Mrs Silver. Her name brings to mind a person who is lovely, soft and sparkly but she was the complete opposite – prickly fierce and scary. She was pencil thin, had jet-black hair and always wore bright-red lipstick, which made her look even more frightening. I remember she wore high heels so you always heard her before you saw her as her feet thundered down the corridor.

As I sit here thinking about her and her English class, I feel sad how quickly time passes. It doesn't seem so long ago that I was sitting in her class with my eyes down reading the text, hoping she wouldn't ask me a question, which of course she always did. It didn't matter because I always knew the answer; I knew the texts inside out, I lived and breathed them. That pleased Mrs Silver; sometimes she looked at me as if her red mouth was actually going to break into a smile.

Many years ago when I was working as a nurse, an actor was admitted to the ward. He told me that I would make a wonderful Lady Macbeth. 'I could just see you playing her,' he told me.

He invited me to come to his evening class at the Birmingham School of Drama. He told me to think about it and gave me his number. I didn't have the confidence to do it; I thought I wouldn't be good enough so I never rang him. But I have always thought it is a wonderful role for any actress.

At the beginning of the play, Macbeth encounters three witches who predict that he will become king. Calamitously, he shares the witches' prediction with his wife, Lady Macbeth, a woman full of lethal ambition. She tells her husband that they must kill King Duncan as soon as the opportunity arises in order for this prophecy to come to fruition. She tells Macbeth to 'screw your courage to the sticking place and we'll not fail'.

Once Macbeth has killed the king, a whole chain of events ensues resulting in murders, madness and suicide. Macbeth repents his heinous crimes, but Lady Macbeth tells him he must not think about it: 'these deeds must not be thought after these ways: so it will make us mad'.

I know that I spend a lot of time ruminating over past events and these are manifested into negative thoughts. This is often the case when you are depressed; in fact, rumination is one of the most problematic cognitive symptoms associated with depression (Nolan-Hoeksema et al, 1999). There is often a self-critical tone to rumination. Lady Macbeth is right in that brooding over past events in a negative way will only compound the situation and not make it better (although murder would be difficult to forget!).

What I am finding so beneficial about my journaling is that it allows me the opportunity to reflect on my past in order to explore and understand myself more and work through my problems. I am clearly still brooding too much on past events that have had a negative impact, but I am hoping the CBT will help me look at the past in a more positive way and view it more with nostalgia.

Interestingly, what follows in the play is Lady Macbeth's swift demise because she cannot stop thinking of what they have done to Duncan: 'Who would have thought the old man to have had so much blood in him?' She constantly sees his blood on her hands and eventually goes insane and kills herself.

When Macbeth finds out she has gone mad, he asks the doctor: 'Canst thou not minister to a mind deceased. Pluck from the memory a rooted sorrow. Raze out the written troubles of the brain?'

I wish there was an eraser that could go into my brain and rub out what feels like nasty, rancid poison. But what has happened has happened, as they say. All we can change is the way we look at it and remember it.

I think in order to look to the future, the past has to be viewed with introspection rather than rumination. Rumination will keep us standing still, firmly in the past and going round in circles or, as I like to call them, ever-decreasing circles. Introspection takes us forward, hopefully to a more positive place.

CHAPTER 22

Daddy dearest

"And when did you last see your father? When he exhaled his last breath? When he last smiled? I've been trying to recall the last time I actually saw him…"
- Blake Morrison, *And When Did You Last See Your Father?*

A woman with dark hair walks past; I have seen her before. She stares in at me and I feel like she is evaluating me as I sit on the sofa writing. She is probably wondering why I am always here.

The phone has rung twice this morning but I didn't answer it. My mum has left a message that she is at home all day; if I want to talk, she is there. I can't ring back, not today. I don't have the strength to talk about how I feel because, if I am totally honest, I don't feel any better. Quite simply, the future still looks bleak. The thought of living seems pointless.

I am sitting here looking at the Christmas tree. Is it really Christmas in a few weeks? I used to love decorating the tree with my dad when I was younger. He loved Christmas, I think because he never had proper Christmases when he was young.

When I was about fourteen, he started to let me have a little drink with him while we decorated the tree. I would stand and sip my Martini and lemonade, feeling extremely grown up, whilst hanging decorations and baubles. Around that time, we started wearing matching outfits at Christmas: matching shirts, bow ties and waistcoats. It was a lot of fun and it made me so happy that my dad and I had this special tradition that was just ours.

After he died, I had a lot of vivid dreams about his hands. I think that was because he used to tickle me when I was little, which I loved, or hold my hand when we were out. When I got older, we used to walk arm in arm.

In one dream, I found out that I was dying from cancer. Dad told me, 'Don't worry, there is nothing to this dying lark.' In my dream I died, and I thought that was fine, it's fine because now I would be with my dad.

As I started looking for him, I got more and more upset because he was nowhere to be found. Then I heard his voice saying, 'I am not really dead, it was all a joke,' and I started screaming and screaming, unable to stop.

The dream seemed so real, and I had it almost every night. My grief seemed endless, with no reprieve, but eventually time moved on and it became less raw. I could focus more on the happy memories.

Eighteen years after his death, and I still remember the excitement he used to get around Christmas. He loved giving out the presents one by one from under the tree on Christmas Day. We sat there and watched each person open their presents, and it used to take hours. I remember the first year I spent Christmas with my husband's family. I couldn't understand why everyone was opening presents at the same time. *That's not how it's done,* I thought.

Since his death, I always dedicate a light of love for him around Christmas time. I go to the cathedral in the city centre, light a candle and read his name in the book of remembrance. I received all of the paperwork for this year but it has remained in my bedside table drawer because I haven't been able to fill it out.

I think about visiting the cathedral and lighting a candle for Dad, but I realise that it won't happen this year and I feel completely hopeless.

CHAPTER 23

Just me and the cats

"One day I was counting the cats and I absent mindedly counted myself."
- Bobbie Ann Mason, *Shiloh and Other Stories*

I read on the internet today that cats are renowned healers, so the fact I am the proud owner of two felines means maybe I am in with a chance of getting better.

I look at my ginger-and-white cat, Sheamus, sleeping on his back. He often stretches out with his tummy exposed, very unlike a cat. He never minds me stroking his belly, which apparently is a sign of complete trust. He stretches out that little bit more when I do it, so I know he likes it. His belly is white and it hangs down when he walks. He reminds me of Bagpuss, all baggy and a bit loose at the seams. He loves nothing more than people fussing him and is soft to his very core.

Now that Sheamus has grown rather rotund due to the fact I can't help spoiling him, he has given up catching birds as he is too slow. He spends most of his time, up to about eighteen hours, asleep. He loves the pillow that I have put down for him in the lounge and sleeps on that most of the time. My husband says he looks like a little prince.

Sheamus's exhaustion today has come from attacking the Christmas tree. I wonder if he dreams. He looks so content lying there; what a wonderful life he has. Thinking that makes me feel happy.

Whenever I stroke my cats, I feel more relaxed. Studies have shown that it releases 'the love hormone' oxytocin in the body, which makes you feel all warm and fuzzy inside. Research suggests this can reduce anxiety.

Aside from this, animals help to prevent loneliness and give unconditional love. The fact that you are caring for another living being stops you thinking so much about yourself, which can often be a good thing. I prefer animals to humans any day – humans are overrated.

I had never owned a cat until I met my husband. He is a great cat lover and persuaded me to have one. Since then, I have never looked back. This is what I love about cats:

- Their whiskers
- Their eyes
- Their different colourings
- Their sweet little faces and ears
- The way they look so serene when they are asleep
- Their purr
- Their aloofness
- The way they rub up against you.

- The way they love a cuddle, if you are lucky like me and have an affectionate one
- The way they wash themselves
- Their agility
- Their dignity
- Their independence
- Their paws
- Their tails
- That they are challenging.
- That they aren't needy

I think I could go on and on, but you get the picture: I LOVE CATS!

As I sit scribbling all of this down, I search on the internet for information about my feline friends.

www.we-love-pets.co.uk tells me that:

A cat purrs within a range of 20–140 Hz which is known to be medically therapeutic for illnesses in humans. A cats purr can not only lower stress it can also help laboured breathing, lower blood pressure, help heal infections and even heal bones...studies have shown and proven that the physical effects are real. If purrs can heal bones, they can positively impact the effects of stress and anxiety. Simply petting a sleeping cat and hearing them purr will help.

The mental health foundation conducted a study with cats protection in 2011 which involved 600 cat and non-cat owning respondents, with half of them describing themselves as having a mental health problem. The survey found that 87% of people who owned a cat could cope with everyday life much better thanks to the company of their feline friends. Half of the cat owners felt that their cats presence and companionship was helpful. Followed by a third of. Respondents who described stroking a cat as a calming and helpful activity.

The company of my cats over the last few weeks has given me so much solace. When I am sitting on the sofa and one of them wants some attention, I only need to feel their soft fur and hear them purr and, in that moment, it is like the sun has come out from behind the dark clouds.

CHAPTER 24

Drowning in a sea of paper

"You deserve a longer letter than this; but it is my unhappy fate to seldom treat people so well as they deserve."
- Jane Austen

I receive a letter today from the CBT service today telling me that unfortunately, due to the waiting list, they are unable to send me an appointment straight away. Reading those words makes me feel lightheaded. I guess I should know that the NHS works at a glacial speed.

They enclose two leaflets with the letter. One is on anxiety (a self-help guide) and one is about panic (a self-help guide) both of which are quite lengthy.

The self-help guides answer questions such as:

1. What is anxiety? *I have a pretty good idea already!*

2. Am I suffering from anxiety? *Grrr!*
3. Causes of anxiety
4. What keeps anxiety going

I skim read the words. In the list of typical experiences of people who suffer from anxiety it says, '*it feels as though something is in my throat. My mouth is dry, and I can't swallow properly and then I begin to get panicky. I think I am going to stop breathing.*'

I think about driving to the post office alone, conversing with the cashier and paying for the Christmas parcels that need to be posted. I feel fear course through my pounding heart to the tips of my toes, and I know with complete conviction that I won't be leaving the house today.

Under the section about what keeps anxiety going, it states that sometimes a vicious cycle develops. Anxious situation – feel bodily symptoms – thoughts that '*something awful is going to happen*' – feel more anxious – thoughts '*now I really am in danger*'.

It goes onto say that: *once a vicious cycle has developed then avoidance is often used as a way of coping ... the sorts of things that people tend to avoid when they suffer from anxiety are most often not real dangers but busy shops, buses, crowded places, eating out, talking to people etc.*

Just reading the information makes me feel breathless. In order to manage my anxiety better, they suggest that I keep an anxiety diary for a period of two weeks and to score it between 0–10.

I feel quite overwhelmed by all of the new information and suggestions, so I know I won't read the panic self-help guide. They will both be put away in my bedside table drawer.

I feel so fearful today. It is Christmas in a matter of weeks; soon it will be January and I know I will feel more pressure to try and get better. People keep telling me to get Christmas out the way first, that the words have become a security blanket. When I think about it being taken away, I feel pure terror. *Anxiety level +100.*

I see Sheamus curled up asleep on the windowsill. I see two robin redbreasts fluttering on the branches. I think about the wonderful text messages from all of the dear people in my life who encourage me to keep going. I want to believe it means something that they care; I want to believe that there is a point to my life. Because, for now, it's eluding me.

CHAPTER 25

Talk is cheap

"I've realised therapy is incredibly therapeutic."
- Lisa Schroeder, *I Heart You; You Haunt Me*

My friend texted me today and said one of her friends, who was diagnosed with breast cancer, was seeing a psychologist. He told her that she was only allowed to spend half an hour thinking about her cancer or looking at things on the internet.

In response to this, I would say that every single person and situation is unique when facing this disease, as is the advice for each individual to deal with it. I am aware that I can't sit on the sofa writing and reading forever – I know that has to stop eventually, or at least take up less of my time. I am sure that continuing in some form (just not as all-consuming) will still be a positive thing to do. The counselling will add a new dimension to my situation, and hopefully enable me to move that little bit further forward.

I have my assessment today at the Link. I can't do this over the phone; it needs to be carried out in person.

I wake up covered in sweat this morning, a pool of water resting between my breasts. My husband and son have left and I feel so alone and desolate, like I am going to sit an exam that I haven't revised for. I am going to sit it in the middle of the city centre with loads of people passing me by, and they will see that my answers are wrong and that I don't know many of them. They will walk away muttering, 'I can't believe she doesn't know the answer to that question. What an idiot. Mind you, what do you expect?'

I want to crawl back into bed until all this is over, but it will never be over unless I take a small step forward. So I stay on the sofa with the leaflet in my hand.

The Link counselling service helps people with a wide range of issues including depression, loss and bereavement, relationship difficulties, abuse, confusion and despair. I read the list and wonder where I fit in. The back page of the leaflet is a green-and-white design. It states that, after the initial meeting, *you will be able to find out whether you think we can help.* I like this wording because there is no pressure to pursue it. It is completely my choice. It goes on to say: *Once you start your sessions with a counsellor, you may expect to see them for as long as you both feel it is of benefit.*

My father-in-law arrives to pick me up. I feel so vulnerable, but I know that if I don't go it is like admitting that I don't want to get better so there is no choice. Not going means I'd be stuck.

My father-in-law parks as close to the building as possible and I manage to walk from the car to the entrance, even though I feel like I am going to be swept away into the void. I don't count steps this time. Am I improving?

The counselling service is on the ground floor of a building named The Sovereign Centre, and I wonder why it is called that. It makes it sound like a bright and friendly place but in reality it reminds me of an old-fashioned dance hall. There are offices all around the edge of the reception area and a table and four chairs in the middle, where you wait to be summoned for your appointment. There are a few magazines to read.

We find the appropriate office and knock on the door to announce my arrival. We are greeted by a lady in her fifties with grey hair and a face that is neither kind nor unkind, just blank. 'I will be carrying out your appointment and I won't keep you long,' she says.

My father-in-law leaves and I sit on the chair to wait, feeling very anxious. I look around and notice a man watching me. He is sitting on a chair on the upper floor above me. I think he realises why I am here. *You've gone a bit crazy, haven't you?* he is thinking.

The counsellor comes out of her office and asks me if I would like a cup of tea. I reply, 'Only if you are making yourself one.' She tells me that she is.

After a while she returns with my tea, and says, 'I don't usually make tea for people.' That makes me feel bad about myself.

I follow her upstairs to one of the small meeting rooms which has three comfy chairs. I am unsure which one to sit on, and I am relieved when I pick the right one.

She begins by asking me questions similar to the ones I have already been asked. 'Have you contemplated suicide?'

It feels pointless to tell her about the tree, so I tell her no, I haven't. My inner voice is saying, *You have to stop thinking about her comment about the tea. You have to NOT THINK ABOUT IT.*

'Have you ever taken an overdose of tablets?' Nope. She looks up from her sheet and gives me a sharp look, so I change my answer to no.

'Have you ever been violent or shown aggression to anyone?' I am sitting placidly in the chair with my hands on my lap. Maybe she thinks I will suddenly produce a weapon from under my jumper and lunge at her. I shake my head. *You don't need to fear me,* I think.

She establishes that I am in no immediate danger and neither are others, so we can move on. 'What has led to your present situation. Why did it start?'

These questions lie heavy in front of me. It feels like concrete has filled my brain. *Oh for goodness sake… It just is…*

I can't make sense of my thoughts but I have to say something. 'Losing my dad. My mum also suffered from cancer some years ago. Pretending in my job, feelings of worthlessness, that I haven't achieved a lot…' I trail off.

She is scribbling away on the piece of paper attached to her clipboard. Am I talking too fast? I feel like I have to fill the air with words then she will be pleased.

Her nodding confirms that this is an all-too-common picture that she has seen before. In a minute she will let out a sigh and think how good it is that people like me exist because I keep her in a job.

She wants to talk about *the trigger*. How it all started. There's quite a long silence… I tell her about a friend who died a year ago in tragic circumstances. Maybe that was it? He was more than a friend really, he was my first love. Could that have been the trigger?

The counsellor is writing it all down. She seems pleased that her A4 sheet of paper is getting filled in. I want to run away and keep looking at the door, wondering if I could excuse myself and leave. But of course I don't.

The session moves on. 'Would you be happy with a student counsellor?' she asks me.

I reply quite forcefully, 'No, I wouldn't!' The counsellor looks a bit startled. 'I am sorry if that sounded a bit harsh,' I say, 'but no.'

'They have had three years' experience. They aren't youngsters. Most of them are in their forties. Many of us have had other careers before doing this, so we all have a lot of life experience,' she says.

'What did you used to do?' I ask her.

'I couldn't possibly answer that. I don't talk about that with clients,' she tells me firmly.

She hands over the counselling agreement for me to read. It contains things such as code of conduct and confidentiality. It tells me that the sessions will be fifty minutes in duration, but if I arrive late my session will be shorter. It tells me that I have six sessions and then both my counsellor and I should know if I need six more. It tells me that the Link is a non-profit making charity; they suggest a donation of up to forty pounds a session.

She hands me a small brown envelope for my donation to give to my counsellor at my first session. I need to take the form away and sign it, and then my counsellor will sign it as well. She says the envelope is sealed and anonymous, so no one will know the amount I put in it. I put both in my bag, knowing they are both useless to me.

It is finished. She has completed her forms, lists and tasks. She has the same blank look on her face that she had at the start. She has made me feel on edge, unwelcome and almost a hindrance. It could be my paranoid mind, but I need a sign from her that she acknowledges the effort and strength it has taken for me to be here today. But there is nothing.

She walks me to the front entrance. 'There isn't a long waiting list so you should hear in January.' Before I can respond, she turns back to her office.

I assume she will go via the kitchen to make herself another cup of tea. As she makes it, she will think she has done a really good job. She will wonder briefly about me; she may ask herself, 'God, what is the matter with these people?' By this afternoon, she won't even recall my face or name. She has met countless people like me and she will meet countless more. Most of them will be forgotten. But we clients will remember her blank face, her curt comments, remember how she made us feel bad about ourselves.

When I am safely back home, I write this all down in my pink notebook and wonder if it could all be in my mind. Maybe I'm judging her unfairly and she was actually perfectly nice. But I didn't feel any sort of empathy or warmth from her.

I have to go with my instincts and I know that even walking through that door again would be impossible. For the time being, I will carry on with my own therapy and hope the CBT will be more successful.

CHAPTER 26

The power of the written word

"The written word endures, the spoken word disappears."
- Neil Postman

I sit in my usual spot on the sofa thinking about the Christmas presents that still need posting, the hoovering that I need to do. The kitchen floor is filthy and dust has settled in the bedrooms upstairs. It makes me feel weak. I don't have the strength to do any of it ... just to write.

Is it helping? I doubt myself today. I look up some information on journaling on my friend Google. A lot of the sites say that journaling can definitely help with mental health, so that is heartwarming:

Journaling requires the application of the analytical, rational left side of the brain; while your left hemisphere is occupied, your right hemisphere (the creative, touchy-feels side) is given the freedom to wander and play (Grothaus, 2015) Allowing your creativity to flourish and expand can be cathartic and make a big difference in your daily well-being.

It's hypothesised that writing works to enhance our mental health through guiding us towards confronting previously inhibited emotions (reducing the stress from inhibition. Helping us process difficult events and compose a coherent narrative about our experiences. (Baikie and Wilhem, 2005)

But I do wonder if pouring out all my past history, failings and mishaps is not going to be effective if it is not done in the right way. I need to find out more.

I find a site www.journal therapy.com that describes a set of guidelines to follow when writing in a journal:

*1. **W–What** do you want to write about? What's going on? How do you feel? What are you thinking about? What do you want? Name it.*

*2. **R–Review** or **reflect** on it. Close your eyes. Take three deep breaths. Focus. You can start with "I feel…" or "I want…" or "I think…" or "Today…" or "Right now…" or "in this moment…"*

*3. **I–Investigate** your thought and feelings. Start writing and keep writing. If you get stuck or run out of ideas, close your eyes and re-centre yourself. Re-read what you've already written and continue writing.*

*4. **T-Time** yourself. Write for 5–15 minutes. Write the start time and the projected end time at the top of the page.*

*5. **E-Exit** by re-reading what you've written and reflecting on it in a sentence or two: "As I read this, I notice…" or "I'm aware of…" or "I feel…" Make a note of any action steps to take.*

It is reassuring to see that what I have been doing is effective to a certain degree. I focus on the phrase 'action steps'. That's the hardest part, not just taking a step but making a positive one. I will need the CBT to help me with that. The journaling alone, just like the medication, is not going to be enough for me.

There is loads of evidence on the internet that confirms how journaling helps sufferers identify and accept their emotions. It is not a substitute for treatment but it is a good complement to other treatments. If you have mild depression then it can work on its own.

I find the journaling:

1. Gives me something to focus on.

2. Helps me to stay calm.

3. Helps me identify my thought patterns and my self-awareness.

4. Gives me some control over what feels like a hopeless situation.

5. Brings me some perspective.

In general, people diagnosed with major depressive disorders report significantly lower depression scores after three days of expressive writing, twenty minutes per day. (Krpan, Knossos, Berman, Deldin, Askren and Jonides, 2013)

The fact that I am writing nearly every day for around four-and-a-half hours should be doing me good. I wonder if I had an MRI scan on my brain it would be packed full of hippopotamuses?!

CHAPTER 27

One small step

"It is a far, far better thing that I do, than I have ever done; it is a far, far better rest I go to than I have ever known."
- Charles Dickens, *A Tale of Two Cities*

I am starting to do inconsequential things like hoovering and dusting. I feel like I am seeing things differently. The Christmas tree looks prettier and offers me more pleasure when I look at it. Am I getting better? Is my brain repairing slowly? I am starting to see a point to things like the flowers that a friend brought me, recognising the subtle pink colour of the lilies and enjoying them. I experience a feeling I haven't had for such a long time ... contentment.

I have been on the 100mg of sertraline for two weeks now and it is clearly working. Yesterday I managed to walk back from my mother-in-law's house on my own. She walked part of the way with me. Once I was alone, my legs felt like they were wading through thick mud and I could hear my breaths. The sound seemed to thunder in my ears; my breaths were so shallow and small that they left me lightheaded. I only walked alone for about five minutes but, once I was back home and the door was locked, I felt exhausted but proud of myself.

A few days later, I actually manage to drive my car. I haven't driven for a month and decide that today I will pick my son up from school. I have Radio Two on and, as I'm listening to Christmas songs and singing along (yes, actually singing!), I feel a connection with life, my life. As I wait for my son, I am so relieved to be alive and so thankful that my health is improving.

It feels like such a good day today; even the sun is shining. I still haven't heard about an appointment with the CBT service which I desperately need because I am undoubtedly still ill. The journaling is continuing, the researching and reading my faithful books. As the weeks have gone by, I realise that I have so much love surrounding me. I am seeing that more clearly now.

My mind continues to consist of two opposing sides. One side wants to believe that I can move forward and the other side is pulling me back, whispering in my ear that I am still a worthless person who doesn't deserve to live a full and happy life. I continue to feel out of place and disassociated from my surroundings, but perhaps that will always be the case. The daily discomfort in my chest reminds me that I am mortal and one day all of this will be over, so I know I have to treasure what I have

I am certainly at a crossroads. This next part of my life will have to be different. My friend asked me what I was going to do with the last half of my life. She certainly knows how to make someone with depression feel good!

Although I have maintained the same routine for a long time, and despite it not bringing me any real joy, I have continued doing it as that is the easier option. I know that for some people routine is comfortable but, although I have to follow certain routines, for my own sake I will have to make some small changes.

I remember in *Hamlet* the quote: 'there is nothing good or bad but thinking makes it so.' Hamlet spends most of the play deliberating over whether to avenge his father's murder at the hands of Claudius, his uncle, and it is his inaction that leads to a string of tragic events. Thinking: where does it get you? Hamlet believes he is more of a thinker than a man of action, but it's the constant thinking that can be self-destructive.

As I sit here now and hear the clock ticking loudly, I know that once I feel better I will have to take some sort of action and not just be stuck. Nothing drastic, just start with small steps.

Not long until Christmas now. This morning the alarm didn't go off, so it was a rush. Christmas jumper day today for both my son and husband. My son appears wearing his blue one that has a snowman with an orange carrot for a nose. Today his teacher will let them do colourings of Santas and such like. I watch him go into school to meet his friends, so full of anticipation and excitement.

Sheamus is asleep on the rug and Cleo is outside. Her incontinence is getting worse. I came down this morning to a river of urine in the kitchen. If that had happened a week ago I would have been anxious about the disruption to my routine, but now if my routine is disjointed it's okay. I am even spraying myself with perfume.

I am starting to feel like my old self, but the fight inside me continues and it seems relentless. Will it ever cease?

My neighbour has taken in my dustbin again. Seventy-four steps would be easy now. Remembering how hard that was just a few weeks ago is painful, but I realise that I have come a long way in a very short space of time.

Sheamus wakes up and contemplates leaping onto the Christmas tree from the sofa. He realises that he is too heavy so begins pawing the baubles before getting tired and flopping onto the wooden floor and showing me his white belly.

The Christmas tree has some new lights because half of the old ones failed to work yesterday. The only ones left in the supermarket were red berry ones, more appropriate for Halloween. I think they look hideous but my son thinks they look *groovy!*

How do I feel looking at the tree with all of the presents underneath? I think nostalgic is the word. I have lined up all my Penguin Classic clothbound books that I have collected over the years on top of the radiator cover. They look good and seeing them makes me feel like me again.

Yes, today is definitely a good day. I am having more of these, and I am starting to look forward to things more. My husband is out tomorrow on his work's Christmas night out. I am invited, but that is a step too far for me at the moment. I will get into my Christmas pyjamas and watch my box set. I am going to enjoy that.

Soon I will make a proper lunch, not just crackers, and watch the Christmas film that I videoed yesterday. I am improving. How I will feel in January I don't know. The security blanket of Christmas will be gone. New Year 2016: what will it bring for me? It is going to be one small step at a time, small steps forward and small changes to my life, then everything else should follow.

I am using everything to try to move forward: medication, love, journaling and even my cats!

CHAPTER 28

You only get one mum

"Whatever else is unsure in this stinking dunghill of a world, a mother's love is not."
- James Joyce, *Portrait of the Artist as a Young Man*

Someone said to me once, 'You only get one mum.' I was young then and probably rolled my eyes. My mum was just *so* annoying, but aren't all mums to a certain extent? I hear my son say it quite a lot, 'Mum, you are so annoying,' as he flounces upstairs to his room and slams his bedroom door shut.

One day in 2004 that phrase came back to me brutally. My mum had cancer and it was very serious; the consultant thought it might be pancreatic cancer. When I saw her in the hospital bed with her skin a horrible yellow colour, she said bluntly, 'They said that with a tumour this big, I should be dead.' She will always be one of the bravest people I have ever known.

I remember sitting outside the hospital on the grass with the summer sun on my face and feeling like I didn't belong to the world. Everyone kept telling me, 'You must be brave.' I wanted to scream at them to let me breathe for a moment, to let me feel... I remember thinking, *please don't let anything happen to my mum, I just couldn't bear it*. How would I function?

I remember helping her to wash her hair in the hospital shower, watching her rinse it and then cup some water in her hands to wash her yellow skin. The sight pulled at my heart strings. When I had helped her back into bed, she told my sister and I that, if anything happened to her, she wanted us to enjoy our lives. She said she could feel Dad with her, calling her. If it was pancreatic cancer, that was the way it was meant to be. See what I mean about brave?

When you are faced with a situation that could take your mum away from you forever, the memories you bring to mind are the ones that you thought had long been forgotten. Meaningless events at the time, but now so poignant. You come to the realisation that most of your childhood memories are centred around your mum – the children's TV programmes you watched together, the afternoon teas of sandwiches and cakes she'd have waiting when you got back from school.

I remember the times she bathed my scraped knees or pulled thorns out of my arms when I had fallen off my bike in the garden into the rosebush. I remember the tears in her eyes when I left for Australia for a year, the dance recitals and school concerts where I would look into the audience and be reassured that she was always there. She never missed a single one. She's my mum and the ties that bind us are strong.

A few days later, my sister and I were walking her dog in the park. We sat on a bench that read: *In memory of... The greatest gift in life is to love and be loved.* We watched an old couple walk by holding hands. My sister asked me why our parents couldn't have had that.

'I understand what you mean,' I said. 'But for all we know there may be some tragedy that couple are dealing with. We have no idea what horrors other people may be facing.'

In the hospital, Mum chatted away to the patients around her. The woman in the bed opposite had died and a new lady was already there. Little Elsie in the corner bed was all bent over with osteoporosis; she had a little voice that reminded me of the mice in *Bagpuss*. Joan in the bed next to mum had stomach cancer and looked pale and transparent. Her eyes were already becoming vacant, life ebbing out of her. All this suffering in one single room. There are times when life just makes no sense.

The day my mum's results arrived, my sisters and I were summoned into the consultant's office. I remember sitting there thinking how strange that in these terrible situations someone knows your own destiny before you do. Who said we have control over our lives? We don't really; we are just tiny specks in a vast universe.

The small room was really hot and I felt the sweat dripping down my forehead. When the doctor told us the results, we all hugged and cried. Mum didn't have pancreatic cancer, she had lymphoma – the same cancer that had killed my dad. It was still cancer, but at least we had a fighting chance.

The haematologist said it was bad luck that we were here again, but lymphomas are becoming more and more common. Mum was to have six months of intense chemotherapy with six injections every three weeks, eighteen injections in total. She was told that she would feel ghastly and lose all of her hair. The truth was that they didn't know if she would get better, they just hoped that she would.

I remember Mum saying with real conviction, 'I will do whatever is needed.'

The next day, my sister and I went to the library to get books out on lymphoma and nutrition and we came across one about a man who had beaten cancer three times. He had had leukaemia and the doctors had told him he only had months to live; twelve years later he was still around. A miracle.

There was a chance that Mum could get better, and she certainly had the mindset to do it. Like that man had written at the front of his book, *Where there is hope there is life.* Mum had all of her treatment and embraced everything, even losing her hair. She got some lovely colourful floppy hats to wear. With the amazing medical team, her pure tenacity and the love of her family, she got well again.

Today I feel hopeful; tomorrow I may not, but today I do. It is a good day. I am alive and should be thankful for that, as so many people are not. They would tell me not to waste my life because it is a precious gift. I just have to have the strength to believe that.

I recall Wendy in the bed next to my mum, who was in her late thirties and had been diagnosed with breast cancer that had spread to her bones. She had endured an abusive marriage and finally found the strength to leave her husband. She had happiness in her life with her new partner who, she told us, was the love of her life. I remember her on the day she was waiting for the results to see if the cancer had spread to her brain. She will be long gone now. I hope she was surrounded with love at the end. Today, I can believe that she was.

I remember Mum telling me once that she was enjoying her treatment because she was experiencing something different. Only she could see it that way! She is a true inspiration.

My friend has just rung to ask if she can come round to see me later. I even feel like watching another Christmas film with my lunch. I still exist. There is still hope and that is all I need to hold on to.

CHAPTER 29

And finally ... CBT

"Anointest my head with conductant. Do I get a crown of thorns?"
- Ken Kesey, *One Flew over the Cuckoo's Nest*

Christmas is now a distant memory and today is the day that I have my first cognitive behavioural therapy session. I am now functioning on some level, thanks to my husband, my son, friends, books, journaling and medication. I can leave the house, although I still feel the fear nagging at me, waiting in the wings to say, 'Come on in, it's your turn again.'

How do I feel today? Obviously nervous, but pleased that the day is finally here. It's like I am stepping into the 'mind the gap' bit of life, hoping that it can start to be filled and stay filled. The constancy of feeling okay is what I crave.

I take myself to my appointment as the hospital is only a mile up the road. Parking is fine, which is one hurdle completed. It still feels strange being outside, and for now it remains an alien and unfamiliar place.

Once I am in reception, I am directed to the waiting area. It is a light, bright, carpeted area which is very pleasant. I see people wandering about and watch them intently, wondering which one might be my counsellor. The magazines on offer hold no appeal so I sit staring into space. To think that only a short time ago that wait would have been agony, but now it is bearable.

Eventually my counsellor appears and introduces herself. My first impression of her is that she is attractive, calm and softly spoken. She leads me to a cosy room with cream walls and flowers in vases. I take a moment to catch my breath as she begins 'the housekeeping' that she needs to do.

As I sit on the small cream sofa and she sits on the chair opposite me with bits of paperwork in front of her, I feel like I have found a safe haven, a place where I can sit and talk to a person who is not going to judge, criticise or offer platitudes, but solutions.

I looked again at the NHS website before my appointment so that I was prepared. I understand that the goal of CBT is to break the cycle of negative thoughts, as they often affect behaviour and feelings. It works by looking at different situations that you may find yourself in, what thoughts and feelings you might experience and how they could impact your behaviour. CBT helps to identify negative thought patterns and looks at ways to try and restructure them to be more positive. I realise that there will be a discussion around my specific problems and I will have goals that need to be achieved. CBT focuses on how you think and act now, rather than attempting to resolve past issues.

My counsellor tells me that each session will last for around forty-five minutes. She recommends starting with six appointments and then reviewing. Today's session involves a lot of questioning about me, my background, my feelings and what has happened in my life to bring me here. Then she explains how she is going to work with me to find solutions to my current challenges. She tells me that I will have homework to do.

As the sessions progressed, the counsellor asked me to keep a thought diary so that any negative thinking styles and patterns could be identified. I shared some very deep personal experiences, which I wouldn't be comfortable sharing outside that little room, but here is a more light-hearted entry in my thought diary that I will share to give an idea of how CBT works.

The first thing to identify is the situation when these thoughts occurred.

What was the situation?

I picked my son up from school today and, instead of waiting in the car as usual, I stood at the school gates. I don't usually like doing this because there is always a gathering of parents chatting and laughing. I was standing alone and felt so out of place. Their voices seemed so loud. I hated it and felt uncomfortable, like everyone was looking at me.

What were your feelings?

Emotional:

I feel worthless

I think that I have no friends here. Why is that?

Why am I like this?

I must be unapproachable

Physically:

Feel uncomfortable

Embarrassed

How did those feelings impact your behaviour?

I avoided eye contact with people

Stayed in the car the following day

Irritable with my son when he came out of school

Discussion in session:

Challenging the idea that these thoughts may not be completely accurate

Need to notice any unhelpful thinking styles such as:

1. It's always going to be that way

2. It is unlikely to change

3. I am always going to feel worthless

Which belief is most connected to your emotions?

Answer: I feel worthless

Now we need to look for evidence that supports that belief or negates it.

FOR:

I've always felt like this and it has never improved

Haven't seen any change

AGAINST:

Sometimes I don't feel like this

For example, some days when I am standing alone at the school gates, I don't feel so bad about myself

Occasionally someone will chat to me

Evaluation:

We identified that on some days I feel more hopeful and better about myself, therefore the more balanced belief would be that I won't feel worthless all of the time.

How much would that more positive feeling impact your life?

1. I wouldn't feel worthless all the time.

2. I may make a new friend if I try and stand at the gates every day.

3. Wouldn't feel useless.

4. I would feel like I had achieved something.

5. Nothing really bad is going to happen, even if I am always standing alone.

The diary enabled me to identify my thought patterns and their impact on my behaviour. Trying to alter my thought processes to be more positive was both challenging and exhausting. Often I'd sit there and think it was a pointless exercise because things were never going to get any better, but other times I was more positive and felt like I was progressing well. When my six sessions were completed, the counsellor discussed the idea of carrying on independently as she was pleased with how far we had come.

If I am honest, it remains a challenge every day to break those cycles of negativity because the thoughts are deep rooted and many of them go back to my childhood. Trying to keep control of them is beyond hard; some days they are overwhelming, and I can hear my inner voice saying, 'Just give up because you are never going to win this battle'. But then I think of what I've been through, what I've learnt and what I've achieved, and I know in my heart what I have to do. And that is to keep going.

CHAPTER 30

Reflections in 2021.

"I used to think that somewhere along the line, I'd find the key to that perfect life ... and that once I had it, every day would be golden and easy, and everything would fit. But life isn't like that."
- Kristen Higgins, *If You Only Knew*

Hello Reader,

All these years after that terrible time and I still ask myself: am I better? That's the million-dollar question, isn't it? I think the honest answer is I will always be a work in progress. Definitely I have been changed by what happened. Even though it was a relatively short and intense period of time, there is no doubt that it took its toll on me. I don't know whether I will ever truly be the same again but, as someone rather kindly once said, 'You will be you again, just a stronger better version.'

A lot has happened in these five years to test my mental health and there has been a lot of heartbreak, loss and challenges to overcome. But in between life's struggles there have been those little gold nuggets of joy, just like my dad said.

Now, even though my life is far from perfect, the way I look at it has changed. I value it more – my health, my friends and my family. I tell people I love them more; I hug more, I notice things more and I treasure things more. The things that are important are to love and to be loved. I have loved and been loved; I have love and I am loved. That love might not be earth shattering or what I was expecting, but I have it in abundance and it is golden.

So, here are some reflections to ponder on and hopefully take heed of:

1. The wonder of nature can lift your heart so notice it. Take a breath and really LOOK.

2. Don't be too hard on yourself. Everyone slips up and struggles at times, but things will improve with time.

3. Try to not look back too often but, if you do, look back with happiness.

4. Laughter really is good medicine.

5. Smile even when you don't want to; it does help.

6. Kindness never goes out of fashion.

7. Good friends are worth their weight in gold. Keep them close.

8. You only ever get one mum; cherish her.

9. Exercise in some form; it works.

10. Travel and broaden the mind.

11. Whatever job you do, do it well and be proud.

12. Smile at strangers; you never know what they are going through.

13. A cup of tea really can comfort you.

14. If anyone makes you feel bad about yourself, or uses your depression against you, let them pass you by. They are not worth your time.

15. Time heals most things.

16. Step out of your comfort zone from time to time and you will surprise yourself.

17. You really can be stronger than you ever thought possible.

18. Sometimes bad things happen for no reason, so don't try to understand them.

19. Read some books. It doesn't matter what they are. Books are a precious gift that you don't want to miss out on.

20. And finally … you really can never have too many cats! Trust me, they will make you feel good, so get one!

CHAPTER 31

My room with a view

"And all the lives we ever lived and all the lives to be are full of trees and changing leaves."
- Virginia Woolf, *To the Lighthouse*

I have lived in the same house for fifteen years and I feel lucky that my lounge overlooks a row of trees instead of a row of houses. Sitting there, I can watch squirrels scurrying up the trees, I can see birds with twigs in their mouths flying off to add to their nests, and I can hear the birds singing to each other. It is quite special.

My cats love stalking the bushes and can spend hours staring at them, hoping that a treat will somehow magically appear. Being able to see the trees and some of nature really helped me during my illness, and I found them healing and soothing to watch. I think trees are like a comfort blanket; they are wonderful and certainly magical.

Long after we've departed this world, trees will still remain. I think that is very reassuring in itself. Because you admired and appreciated them, it means that you lived, you existed – and therefore you mattered.

THE COMFORT TREE
BY BECKY POWELL

The tree outside my window isn't oak or elm or beech,

It's a comfort tree with wisdom, and the ability to teach,

It's leaves burst full of magic,

That light up in the breeze,

Bringing comfort, warmth and joyful peace,

Through the grace and beauty in its leaves.

The tree outside my window isn't willow, ash or pine,

It's a tree that holds the memories of lives like yours and mine.

The memories of the people that laughed and cried and sighed,

The branches a reminder of their sad and happy times,

Moments quick forgotten through the passing of the years,

The comfort tree a symbol of all their hopes and dreams and fears.

BIBLIOGRAPHY

Primary texts:

I know Why the caged bird sings. Maya Angelou. Virago Press 2007

Jane Eyre. Charlotte Bronte. The Penguin Group 1996

Rebecca. Daphne Du Maurier. Pan Books 1975

The Yellow Wallpaper. Charlotte Perkins Gilman. Penguin Classics 2015

To The Lighthouse. Virginia Woolf. Wordsworth Editions 1994

Macbeth. William Shakespeare. Wordsworth Editions Ltd 2005

Hamlet. William Shakespeare. Wordsworth Editions Ltd 2002.

The Oxford Compact English Dictionary. Oxford University Press 1996.

Websites:

Davey, M 30/6/2015. *Chronic depression shrink the brains memories and emotions*. www.theguardian.com

NHS www.nhs.uk

Kings fund writers, n.d. *Has the government put mental health on an equal footing with physical health?* www.kingsfund.org.uk

MIND www.mind.org.uk

Staff Scientists of Cambridge Brain Sciences Blog, 14/11/2017. *Exercise Increases the size of your hippocampus.* www.cambridgebrainsciences.com

We Love Pets Team, n.d. *Are cats good for our mental health?* www.we-love-pets.co.uk

Nolan-Hoeksema, S. et al. September 2008. *Rethinking Rumination.* www.pubmed.ncbi.nlm.nih.gov

Grothaus,M. 29/01/2015. *Why journaling is good for your health.* www.fastcompany.com

Krpan, K.M. et al. 2013. *An everyday activity as a treatment for depression: The benefits of expressive writing for people diagnosed with major depressive disorder.* www.sciencedirect.com

Baikie,K. Wilhelm,K. 2005 *Emotional and Physical Health Benefits of Expressive Writing.* www.positivepsychology.com

Adams,K n.d. *It's Easy to W.R.I.T.E.* journal.therapy.com

Printed in Great Britain
by Amazon